Has the Lady Been Yet?

By
Kit Derrick

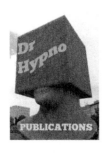

ISBN

Paperback   9781838426798

https://www.facebook.com/Hypnopub

Cover by BLUSH

Acknowledgements

Huge thanks to Jayne Bryson for her wonderful assistance, as always, for correcting my manuscript when the words tumbling out exceeded my ability to spell or punctuate. Any errors that remain are my own fault, as I'm stubborn.

There are two 'thank you' acknowledgements that can never be enough, so I'll leave them simple here.

Thanks to everyone who helped look after and care for Mum; everyone who knew her, and loved her. They know who they are.

Special thanks to my sister, without whom I'd have gone (even more) insane as we went through these experiences; for being there, for sharing and supporting, and for giving her blessing to this project.

Contents

What The Hell Is This book?..1

Intro (Summer 2021) 5

Third Anniversary (Summer 2022) 11

Early Memories of Mum, and Early Signs............................14

In The Meantime 26

Our Indestructible Mum...33

The Dementia Itself...52

The Diagnosis 63

Carers and Caring 82

The Experience - The Funeral 96

The Experiences - Vignettes...103

The End 143

Fiction...149

    Reflections...151

    The Empty Shell...153

    The Empty Shell pt.2 (Self Pity).. 154

    Mum Hated the Dentist..155

    Snapshots.. 157

    Has The Lady Been Yet?... 159

Closure 175

    The Cricket Pitch.. 175

Afterword..177

What The Hell Is This Book?

A good question, thank you for asking. I'm not entirely sure what the answer is myself, and I'll admit that this might be a very strange beast of a narrative. What follows can't be called an instruction manual, isn't meant as a traditional biography or memoir, and it isn't really intended as a self-help book. I think it's just something that needs to be written down and is a story that some people might appreciate reading. I suspect that if the content chimes it will find its own audience, without the need for a genre or definition.

If that seems a strange way to open my book then I'd agree, but once I'd decided that I should put this history down on paper (or computer in my case), I found that I didn't have a clue how to begin, so the title of this prologue is the very question I asked myself. What the hell is this book? Traditionally, and especially with more formal writing, received wisdom is that you should complete all the content and then come back to write your introduction at the very end, when you have a clear overview and are able to neatly combine the themes and experiences into a tidy package, to ease your readers into the subject matter which follows. Somehow, that didn't seem appropriate, so I decided to 'wing it' instead. After all, winging it is what we

1

had to do throughout Mum's illness. The result is the stream of consciousness explanation you're now reading.

What's that? Oh, you actually meant what the hell is the book *about*? Well, that's a little simpler to answer. This book will follow the insidious effects of dementia on a parent and explain the impact on the adult children who watched, cared, tried to assist, and felt frequently helpless as events unfolded beyond their control. As I discovered the hard way, there isn't an instruction manual for this kind of experience, and I'm not arrogant enough to attempt to provide that here. What the words *will* hopefully provide is an insight into my own journey and its lingering after-effects, and the book might help some others prepare, just a little, for the day they might find themselves in a comparable situation. And the story will hopefully show that there can be hope, beauty, and even the occasional humour, in the darkest paths of experience.

There were the worst of times and there were better, occasionally quite wonderful, times over the course of Mum's illness (to badly misquote Dickens), and I intend to share my own reactions to, and feelings about, what happened on our journey too, as painful as this will sometimes be to admit. It may prove cathartic for me, but might also help you to understand what a friend or acquaintance of yours in a similar situation could be going through beneath the surface; what they might really be feeling beneath the façade of coping, despite the fact they tell you that everything is okay. Wow, I'm really not selling this as a fun read, am I? Let me try one more time. This is the book I wish I'd been able to read when Mum had her diagnosis, of someone plainly and honestly talking about what happened to them and what it was like, the good and the bad, and showing that at the end of it all, most of the enduring memories are still positive ones. Despite the fact that this book is ultimately about the death of my mum, I want you to know that it's possible to come to terms with, and accept, that loss, and still keep those special and loving memories at the forefront of everything. It isn't easy, but it's possible.

There are certain events and specifics which are important to Mum's story but which won't be included on these pages, and the truth behind that choice is that some events are not mine to share. Finding that balance between what to include and what to leave out is difficult. My rule of thumb for inclusion will be, "would Mum have been able to see the funny side, or appreciate what was being written?" And if I think she would, and it isn't someone else's pain or reaction, I'll include it. This is, after all, Mum's story as much as mine, so her reactions and sensibilities need to guide me.

I'm fighting against my natural inclination to try and make the writing tidy, literary, and perfect (some hope!), and have opted for a more conversational tone throughout. I hope you don't mind this approach, but I thought it might help you get closer to my own thoughts and feelings, my doubts and struggles in coping, and my own nature, just a bit more fully and personally. So apologies to any grammar or structure fairies who like their reading matter precise and tidy, but dementia isn't about tidiness, perfection, or events unfolding as you expect; that's why this approach also seemed fitting.

As I don't know how to categorise this tome, perhaps I should just describe it for you instead? The text will be split into two distinct parts. The first and main section will be absolute fact (as I remember it), following the journey of discovering, coming to terms with, and dealing with Mum's dementia. The latter part will be what I'd call informed fiction, where I can reveal more of the emotional impact, my fears and thoughts, and my reactions to what happened during the last few years of my mum's life. I can let myself be more open there, free from the conventions of a timeline. In essence, I think the whole book will be best described as a collection of experiences.

These opening paragraphs are the first things I've written down and intended to publish, and are a work in progress. I'd describe myself as a work in progress too. I'm still trying to work out what I actually need to write down, create, and share, in order to make this useful to a reader, and at the same time to form a part of my ongoing healing process. It's more than a little scary to open up about something as personal and devastating as this, as you'll not only learn about my mum, but also get a peek into how my mind works too. You lucky sod.

So I shall take a deep breath, gird my loins, and begin. I hope you find something helpful in what follows.

Intro (Summer 2021)
(From my first handwritten notes, pretty much verbatim)

Hello. So I decided it was time to finally start writing my story properly tonight, though I've wanted to do it for a while; I've felt like I *needed* to. I don't want to procrastinate too much here about my subconscious motivations as, if there's one thing I've learned in recent years, it's that is that life is too short, too fleeting, and too fragile. And I digress enough when I'm talking, so there's no need to add more here.

Having said that (I told you I digress), one of the main reasons I'm writing this story down now is that I don't want to forget how everything felt at the time. I don't want to wait until my own memory starts playing games, inventing interpretations or 'remembering' things that didn't actually happen. I want to write while everything is still raw. Maybe it's the martyr complex that runs in our family which makes me need to do that, and perhaps I need a little self-flagellation too; to punish myself for not doing enough to help Mum. This isn't self-deprecation, it's simply that, when you lose someone you love over an extended period, and to something like dementia, you always wonder if there's more you could have done. That's just human nature. I hope that writing this will help me exorcise some of those demons. The story won't be strictly chronological, as I don't think things were chronological in Mum's mind at the end, but I don't think that matters in this case. It is each individual moment that matters, not where they occur in a series of events.

Mum died two years ago today, as I'm writing these words, and my driving motivation is that I don't want to forget anything; don't want to forget what happened, but don't want to forget how it *felt* at the time either. It does strike me as more than a little ironic that I don't want to forget to write about dementia.

I'll start as I mean to go on, being as brutally honest as I can. So, here's a horrible and painful truth to start. Mum died, and I'm glad that it happened how and when it did.

No, not happy; that's the wrong word (and nuance of language is especially important here, I think). What I probably mean is that I'm glad; glad that Mum died before COVID happened, and glad that she wasn't on her own at the end, glad that our last interactions made us smile. At the same time, her death left a huge Mum-shaped hole in my life, and I suspect that will always be there.

I'll try to explain why I say I'm glad. These last two COVID years would have been absolutely horrific for my mum, and she wouldn't have been able to cope, or to understand what was happening; I know that she wouldn't. And I couldn't bear the idea of seeing her in distress like that. Sometimes, over the past couple of years, I haven't been able to stop myself imagining what that other life might have been like for her, particularly when I heard accounts of families being separated, elderly relatives and patients unable to see their loved ones, and the worsening of their conditions which resulted. My heart goes out to those people, but their stories just re-enforced my belief that Mum going when she did was the right thing; for her, at least.

Things were physically difficult for Mum in the . months, and she was clearly deteriorating from the dementi. too, much as I liked to pretend that she wasn't. Sometimes, I'd create unrealistic fantasies that she'd find a way to miraculously recover, but I knew deep down that it was only a matter of time. Even if that mental deterioration hadn't continued, Mum was already at the stage where some everyday tasks could be daunting or confusing, and if she'd lived on into the COVID times, critical needs like the distancing restrictions, remembering to wash her hands frequently, to wear a mask, or to understand why some people couldn't visit, would have been beyond her. That added stress and confusion would just have accelerated her decline, and would have made her last months unbearable, both to live and to see.

It may sound selfish, but when she left us, she was still discernibly 'Mum,' if you know what I mean, so dementia hadn't completely stolen her away from us. It *is* selfish, but it feels better to have lost our mum in the way we did, rather than having to see a terrified, increasingly ill, and confused mind in Mum's body. In her own wonderfully stubborn way, I suspect that if she was able to look back on the end now, she'd have been almost mischievously pleased that the dementia didn't get to take her away. To coin a phrase she would sometimes use, "that'll cap the little bugger." The dementia didn't "win" after all.

If Mum had stayed with us for another year (which isn't a given anyway, as she was so susceptible to infection), it would have been almost inevitable that she'd have ended up in a hospital ward, and with visitor restrictions, would have died apart from me and my sister, not really knowing *why* we veren't there with her, or what was going on. And that's without the added challenges of carers, medication and general health in the first days of the pandemic, which would have added significantly to her stress and confusion. So *that's* why I'm glad it happened when it did. And how it did.

It was a very bizarre and disconcerting time for me personally, after she'd gone. Looking after Mum had become a central part of my existence, and with that taken away, I became uncertain of my own role and motivations, and of pretty much everything, to be frank. As the days and weeks passed, and I tried to process and come to terms, I realised that I just didn't know what my own purpose was anymore. There was a huge hole in everything. It took quite a while to adjust. One eventual outcome was that I needed a focus for my energies, and in the past two years I've started writing fiction again, something I always wanted to do. And as I threw myself into that obsessively, it gradually occurred to me that it shouldn't just be fiction I was creating. To close that hole that still existed, I needed to fill it by recording what happened, and exploring the changes in me. I think this particular book (experiment?) will be a good thing to complete, and might be the conclusion of that healing process. Not forgetting, but moving forwards. To some extent, it doesn't matter to me if anyone reads it.

I'm often perceived as a negative person; all our family are (or were). But that's just a trick of perception. Being prepared for the worst isn't the same as revelling in, or enjoying, negativity. And perversely, the experience of

losing Mum ha.
positively than ev ok at other things in life more
outside, of course; I re at you'd know it from the
old bugger. But there is a t dfastly committed, grumpy
is gone, and because of the a to everything. My Mum
long before she died, but the b.. part of her had gone
had Mum in it for 82 years, and He is that the world
almost fifty. As a self-proclaimed m.er in my life for
grateful for that. 's boy, I'm so

I love you, Mum.

A personal dedication to you

Happy Death Day, Mum! You and I can share a dark joke like that, because you'd have appreciated it; understood the gallows humour. And joking makes it less likely that we'll cry.

I think I'm writing partly because you wouldn't have remembered the last years yourself, love, so I also want to remember them for you too. And as we discussed once, so we can remember the good times, both pre- and post-dementia.

I won't include anything I think you would have minded being written. Those things stay in the family. I remember you talking about your own dad in hospital, and how the younger him might have been horrified at his lack of control (and perceived dignity) in his daily life at the end, being cared for like a child, and you said that you were happy (I know, happy is the wrong word again. Relieved?) that he'd reached the stage where he wasn't aware enough to worry

about that. You never ...ached that level of
disorientation, not entir ...sistently. There are some
embarrassing things I ...u wouldn't have minded me
sharing, though, as ...u ...ve giggled about them yourself
if you were able, ...u sometimes did. Dementia is a
strange beast, w...an sometimes leave no indication a
single thing is ... At other times...

I'm not g...to include talk about our family, not even
my sis, bey...references where she's integral to the story.
She has h...own story to know and tell, and it's not my place
to intrude on her memories and thoughts. The same applies
to your friends and the rest of the family. This book is an
exhalation of mine; my memories and reflections on those
last years with you. I'll show my sister before I decide
whether anyone else can see, of course; get her take on it,
and hopefully her approval, as she's affected just as much as
me, but this book isn't specifically our story either. It's about
the bigger picture. It's almost abstract; an example of
someone going through what we did, which might help
others find some comfort, reassurance or hints to help them
cope more easily. At least I hope so. And I think you'd
approve of that.

The last thing you said to us, compos mentis, was "bugger
off, you two." I like that fact very much. xxx

Third Anniversary (Summer 2022)

I hadn't intended to add this additional chapter, but I'm editing and revising today, and it seemed very appropriate that I insert a short extra section, despite the fact that the idea of three introductions seems perverse, overkill, and is probably commercially stupid. But screw it, I don't care. Today is important. Important in terms of the events of this book, but also in terms of the ongoing impact on me. Mum died three years ago this morning.

I could tell you that coping with the anniversary has been easier each year, but that would be a lie and, if anything, it preys on me even more. There was a numbness initially, but I found that as the next years passed, I wanted to remember the good times, but the anniversaries and dates I kept a record of aren't those of the jokes she told, the day trips, the hugs. They're the dates of the appointments, the fall, the operation, the death, the funeral, the scattering of ashes, as those were the details we recorded at the time. I'm still working through my feelings, but what I'd like to be able to do, one day, is replace those landmarks with others; with the last time we said, "I love you," the occasion when we first met the quite possibly insane nonagenarian vicar who performed the service, the time when I put on the cardigan Mum knitted as part of the funeral, the bizarreness of scattering ashes with a spoon, something Mum would no doubt have cackled at wickedly. I'm not there yet, but those are the occasions I want to remember each year, so I just need to pair them up in my own mind with the actual dates.

And each year I want to be able to train myself to recall different things. Not the terror at the phone call about her fall, but the relief that she was smiling and seemed fine when I got there. That we were secretly doing crosswords together in A and E, even though the Sister told us not to. The exact circumstances when I took the photo I love, of Mum fake-scowling in her hospital bed as I put a small plastic cup on her head for a picture. Not the dread she needed an operation but joking with her before she went for the op, and seeing her afterwards, miraculously surviving something we never thought she would. Talking through the music we loved and should use for the wake with my sister, remembering trips and songs, and silly family sayings. Those are the things the anniversaries should be about.

I've spoken to my sister, who I sent a draft to, and she also just gave her approval of what I'm doing. I know it's my story, but that means a lot, and validates what I'm trying to create, persuades me that the writing isn't entirely self-indulgent, and that I've not strayed too far from the truth.

Going through the edit today, I noticed the number of occasions when I stray into digression and repetition, and I've been trying to decide just how many of these occasions I should remove. I've taken out the pointless and accidental repetition, of course, but I'm finding it to be a difficult balance in deciding just how much I should treat this as though it is a professional text to be marketed at a certain demographic and fulfil their expectations about style and content. You shouldn't admit this, of course; the creation of a book is like the clichés about the manufacture of laws and sausages; you don't want to know how they're made. But I always intended transparency and honesty to be at the forefront of this, so I'll err on the side of my authentic voice and stream of consciousness. Similar to my approach to grammar and style, I'll retain a lot of the musings, wanderings and occasional echoes and revisiting of events. Repetition has its place, after all, and as you'll see later on, can also be a very powerful and helpful tool in supporting someone with dementia.

Today there were messages from family and Mum's friends, best wishes and kind thoughts from those who know me well, but to everyone else it's just a normal day. Why wouldn't it be? But for me it's three years since she left us, and I want to remember that landmark, so adding a third introduction today seems apt. I think that's the other reason for this page, so today can also commemorate the time I finished adding new words to this book, and, to fall back on a cliché, so we can close this particular chapter. So it's about time I started the story in earnest. Thank God for that, I hear you think, I hope it isn't all going to be like this! Nope. Next chapter is far more 'normal'.

Early Memories of Mum, and Early Signs

"Behave yourself, or we'll put you in a home!" It was a family in-joke and a saying we'd used for years. It might even have started when Mum was in her fifties, and was usually whispered to her in mock-exasperation as she was being mischievous or rude about something under her breath, often in a public setting. I don't know the exact point at which we refrained from making that joke, but our awareness of Mum's health meant that we stopped saying it long before that outcome might have become a genuine option. Jokes should be funny. And there was a lot of other humour in our lives, so this was a 'joke' we didn't need any more. Mum always provided, both intentionally and unintentionally, plenty to laugh about.

That's the over-riding characteristic of my mum, if I had to pick just one; that she was funny. Wickedly funny sometimes; mischievous, dedicated, loving, wonderful, but most of all I remember funny. I'm so pleased that stayed with her right to the very end, which means that it remains the major part of how I remember her.

One of my earliest recollections of Mum (which I know couldn't possibly be an invented memory from a photo or home cinefilm, as this memory was never captured mechanically) took place on a Saturday morning; must have been about 1975. I would have been four years old, sitting at the kitchen table with a cup of milky coffee, and I know it was a Saturday around that year, as I'd just finished watching *Valley of the Dinosaurs* on BBC1 on the colour TV. In my memory, Mum was doing something mum-esque in the kitchen, maybe baking. She had on a very light blue dress with darker blue patterns; I can picture it vividly. That, and the back of her head. I don't remember what she was doing for certain, that part is invention, but I know that she laughed. I know this has to be a real memory because nothing memorable happened, just me sitting there and smiling because my mum had laughed. I have no idea why. It's an image, a moment of recall, nothing more. They say that you remember more when you move house as a child, and this was before our first relocation, in my first home, in a cul-de-sac in Formby. And strangely, I know I was specifically drinking milky coffee. Not strange because I was so young and drinking coffee (this was the seventies so it hadn't become bad for you yet), but strange because, for the rest of my childhood, I drank tea; didn't drink hot coffee until my teens and didn't like it much even then. I'm still not very keen, to be honest. And I still can't abide coffee flavouring in cake or chocolates to this day (in case you wondered). But I know that, in this particular flashback, I loved warm, milky coffee at the time, had asked for it specifically, and was only allowed it on Saturday mornings (I think). This isn't going to be a biography, and isn't just about all the different reminiscences I have of my mum, which would be rather too self-indulgent, but I just wanted to mention this one specific memory because it's genuinely the earliest, definite image I have of her, so an excellent place to start. And she was laughing.

As people get older, it's natural for their kids to worry about them, and up until her mid-seventies, I'd say, my mum was incredibly energetic, busy, interactive, and needed relatively little worrying about (though of course, being a natural worrier, that would never stop me). To give you an example of just how active and capable she was, when she was 75, Mum and I went on a big day out together (the day after watching the opening ceremony of the Olympic games, if you want specifics). After an evening of TV and mutual bitching about Kenneth Branagh's performance, we got up at 6am, walked into Town to get a steam train from Liverpool to Carlisle for our day out, and had an absolutely wonderful time. An exceedingly long day, busy (and delayed) train, walk around all the sights, shopping, lunch out, the full works. So you understand she wasn't exactly housebound, or limited on what she would, or could, do at that point in time. She'd also frequently get the train on her own to go to Yorkshire to see her family, she was a demon gardener (as a septuagenarian would still climb up ladders to trim 6 ft hedges, to my absolute terror). But by 82, towards the end, she didn't leave the house, or her chair, very often. It was a steep decline. This story is about those seven years, but it's also about the beauty of how the Mum I used to know was still with us, sometimes, right up to the very end. If you're reading this and entering an analogous situation, don't give up hope. Never give up hope.

There are two things that most people never realise about dementia, or only realise when it's too late, or if they talk to one of the amazing support charities. Firstly, when you initially suspect it might be happening to somebody close to you, it's probably already too late for most preventative actions. That's a hard truth, and an unkind fact, but we had to deal with a lot of those. You can't actually tell when it begins, either. At first, you might dismiss memory issues as "just age," or the forgetfulness we all have occasionally, and by the time dementia reaches the stage where you finally need to persuade someone to go for a diagnosis, the chances are that you already know full well what the outcome will be. And it could have been growing worse for a long time, while you did nothing. A remnant of that guilt never goes away, despite the fact it is totally irrational, and any suspicions you might have had would have been almost impossible to predict or act on. So that guilt remains. For me, anyway. You just have to live with it and come to terms with the fact that this self-recrimination comes from a place of love. It exists because you loved someone so much and, even after they're gone, you want to find something or someone to blame, even if it is yourself. As the doctor told Mum at the actual diagnosis, dementia isn't anyone's "fault," it's an illness. But that's just a truthful fact. It doesn't make the emotions and the "what if" thoughts go away.

The second thing you should know is that this illness is such an insidious little bugger, and there isn't an exact moment when someone switches from non-dementia to dementia. It isn't an illness you "catch". And worse than that, the symptoms and progress aren't even a type of gradual change which you can try and monitor. In a day, an hour, even over the course of a few minutes, memories and personalities can come and go; one week the sufferer seems to be perfectly fine and you wonder why you were ever concerned, but suddenly, maybe on a Friday, you might notice several indicators that details are being forgotten, a vagueness or lack of concentration that just doesn't seem right might be on display. But by that Friday evening, the person seems fine again, and you can and do easily dismiss those hours of doubt. There is the added complication that, in the earlier stages, the sufferer is quite probably aware that everything isn't right themselves. They have an illness, but they're not stupid. They may dismiss or ignore symptoms, but after a while they know that they are having more problems with their memory and mood than just simple forgetfulness. And at that stage, when they're aware that something isn't right, and are probably too scared to admit or investigate, those around them don't know how adept the dementia sufferer might be at masking or covering up their problems. I think that was certainly the case with our mum.

Dementia sufferers are excellent fibbers and actors (most of the time), and they've had the slow encroachment of the disease to give them time to practice "covering their tracks," to try and stop their loved ones from worrying or from interfering (however well-meaning that interference might be). Even when the sufferer reaches the stage (and it's horrible to say and admit, but the *relief* of the stage) when most of the time they're not consciously aware of their dementia any more, the practice of covering up symptoms is already so ingrained and automatic for them that it can be incredibly difficult for loved ones or carers to spot specific problems, new symptoms, or times of distress. This was certainly true in the case of Mum, and in the last years it became such an automatic reaction to hide the truth of her condition from us that we never knew for sure when she was having a particularly bad day, or might be struggling to identify key facts or people.

Here's a thought that bothered me for such a long time after she died. It's only looking back afterwards that I realised, but there's a distinct possibility that my mum "faked" even really knowing me on numerous occasions in the last couple of years of her life. I don't want to over-exaggerate, and I don't mean not *recognising* me at all (though that too is terrifyingly plausible), but having observed her interactions with other friends and relations, Mum was certainly capable of appearing as if she had total recall and "faking" conversations. Looking back with the benefit of hindsight (is it a benefit here?), it seems to me that there were at least some exchanges when my mum didn't seem certain "who," exactly, I was. Yes, she knew that I was the friendly, loving, helpful Kit who cared for her, the face she recognised and trusted, but I don't even think she was always certain that I was her son. That's an exceedingly awkward thing for me to admit, and to absorb, but I strongly suspect it to be true, and it is certainly a lingering and haunting conviction I can't shake. Being such a lovely and caring woman, I think that Mum knew I was important to her, and that she knew how important she was to me, and would consequently do anything she could to not upset or worry me, or admit that occasionally, in those latter months, the specifics of my identity might have eluded her occasionally. She would just accept that I was there, that I was someone important, and would act accordingly. For her, that would also have the advantage of not confusing or upsetting herself, in trying to remember exact details she didn't need.

19

It's a horrific thought for a child to have, but one that's come back to me numerous times, made worse by the fact that I wouldn't have been aware of this process in her mind at the time. I might have spent several evenings, and had several conversations with, my mum and been blissfully unaware that she didn't really know quite who I was. It's possible that I might be mistaken in this belief, of course, and that it's the result of that lingering guilt I talked about, but looking back and observing some lack of recognition from Mum with other people she was close to, people she saw regularly, I'd be surprised if it hadn't happened with me too, at least once or twice.

I'll begin my story about the dementia proper with one experience that has stuck in my mind for years now. I don't know the exact month or year it took place, as this was a one-off incident with nothing to date it, but this was the interaction that prompted my first serious suspicion that something out of the ordinary might have been going on with Mum's memory. My sister and I had, by this stage, already commented occasionally on Mum's sporadic forgetfulness, but not in terms of any real concern. It was nothing out of the ordinary most of the time and, to be honest, Mum's forgetfulness then might even have been no more than I'm guilty of myself, but on this one specific occasion, it was a little bit different.

It would have been shortly after the time I mentioned, when we went to Carlisle for the day trip. To set the scene, we were in Mum's kitchen and one of her sisters was visiting. I was buttering the bread for lunch, and Mum was mid-conversation when she looked over, and laughed at my poor marge and knifemanship; the spread being lavishly coated in the middle of the bread, but sadly lacking towards the outside of the slices. "Speedway Bread! That was what your mum used to call that, wasn't it?" I don't know if Mum's sister picked up on that comment, but I did, and studiously ignored it, laughing along with her joke. She meant that the phrase was what my nan (my dad's mum) used to use in reference to unevenly buttered bread, with a dry perimeter 'track' around the outside. I don't know if it was just a simple (if odd) slip of the tongue, or maybe just a muddle in her mind that she might have made that same remark to my dad once upon a time and was parroting an earlier comment. I don't honestly think she believed that I was my dad (who'd died when I was a teenager), even momentarily, but I'll always wonder just a fraction. Wonder whether that was the first solid indication that there was something beyond general old-age forgetfulness? Was this the first real sign? Her first noticeable slip in covering up her own confusion? I'll always suspect. I can't claim to accurately recall every second of a conversation which took place years ago, but when I look back on that moment, I swear that I can remember one of those clichéd beats, half a second of silence after she said that to me, before we all carried on talking, and in my mind, I can't help imagining my mum realising the slip herself, waiting for a comment, and when none came, moving on and assuming (hoping) that no-one else had noticed. That would have been late 2012, I guess, well before there were any serious indications that she had a problem.

In 2014, the first 'big' change in my mum's demeanour came, though this wasn't directly related to her memory. Mum had always been active every day, right up until that date; walking up the road to the shops each morning, talking to everyone who lived along the way, chatting merrily and swapping updates, and stories of children and gardens. Then, one morning after I'd stayed over at her house, she was quite flustered when she got back home from the shops, heading straight to the bathroom with barely a word. Something seemed wrong about it.

Mum would never make a big deal of anything, but after a little cajoling she told me she'd had a little 'accident' on the way back from the shops, after stopping to chat to various people, and obviously leaving it a little too long to make it home and to the bathroom. Trying to laugh and pass events off as inconsequential, she'd awkwardly joked that she'd made it to 77 in full control of herself, which wasn't bad, all things considered. I'd been due to go back to my own home later that Saturday morning and, looking back, I should have handled the situation better and just changed my plans automatically, but she'd initially laughed about her little 'accident,' and I knew she hated making a fuss or having either of her children change what they did, just for her. I had my rucksack ready and coat on and she'd gone noticeably quiet, so I asked if she'd like me to stay until the next day. I was surprised when she answered, putting on a child's voice, "Yes!", like a sulky infant; she was joking, of course, but the fact she made the joke at all was very telling.

I said, "of course I'll stay" and put my bag down, and Mum just called me a "silly sod," and we didn't talk about it again. But I know that fake child's voice; I've used it myself, more than once. When you don't want to admit that you want, or need, something, it's an acceptable, jokey way of letting someone know what's bothering you. I hadn't realised how much the event had shaken Mum. Retrospect is great for spotting indicators you should have noticed at the time (or inventing them, a hazard of reflective guilt), but I've wondered a number of times if this might have been the first sign that Mum was starting to worry about herself for her own sake. She was an incredibly strong, practical woman, could deal with anything, and admitting that she needed me, even in a joke voice was, for me, the start of the role reversal that was to come. I know she'd have fretted about that incident, so I'm glad I could provide some small comfort that day, but there's every chance it forced her to reflect on her general wellbeing, including the forgetfulness she was quite aware of. I was oblivious to any of that, of course. I just assumed, as she'd reluctantly told me about 'the accident,' that she would have told me outright if she was worrying about the broader state of her health. I just assumed it was a one-off incident. After all, these things happen to everyone on occasion.

Mum didn't go up to the shops at all for a while after that. Her trips out were sparse in the following days and weeks, and became the exception rather than the rule afterwards, and only then if repeatedly cajoled to go with me, my sister, or her friend. By the end of that year, Mum's trips out were becoming even rarer, and never on her own I don't think; certainly not to anywhere near the extent she had previously. It's so easy to see the turning points when you look back, not so obvious at the time.

I'm certain now that this was the moment when my mum really lost her confidence, and you can't underestimate how vital that is to wellbeing. The positivity in your own capabilities is as powerful as any medicine. For the first time, she started to dwell on her own health for the future. It's easy to see why. Mum must have hated and feared the idea (and I guess must have fixated on the worry) that a similar 'accident' might happen to her again, in public, and along with it, the possibility of having to show and admit weakness. I think we must have an introspectiveness and paranoia in our genetic makeup within our family, though we all try to project an outward shell of confidence (verging on arrogance for me, as I'm not very good at balance), but that isn't through choice, and worry is exhausting. Mum's trick for dealing with this might have been effective, but it was frustrating, and not exactly helpful.

She made the decision, conscious or not, to avoid obsessing by inventing explanations and solutions, and reality be damned. In this instance, the 'solution' seemed to be a practical one; if she didn't go out at all then she couldn't have another 'accident' *while* she was out, and there wouldn't be a problem to worry about. With that potential future sorted, she could also disregard and ignore whatever health-related cause had scared her to begin with. This was typical Mum. The reason she didn't make it to the bathroom in time could have been a bug she'd had, or something she'd eaten or drunk, or just age, but I don't think she wanted to consider any of those. There was always the danger that investigating might indicate a real problem. And ignoring problems was a far easier way of making them go away.

The reason I'm telling this story at all is as an indication of Mum's approach to all illness or weakness in herself, and this just increased over time. She would pretend things hadn't happened as a coping mechanism, convincing herself that whatever occurred was insignificant, so she wouldn't have to worry about any potential consequences. It's not an unusual coping mechanism, but it does mean that those you love can't know what is going on with your health either, so aren't able to help or intervene. Which may have been part of the point.

It's one of those frustrating ways of the world that in another reality this little interaction between us, of Mum actually admitting she'd wanted me to stay with her a bit longer and the result that I did, could have encouraged her to start being more open with me. Instead it began a pattern of Mum automatically denying her illnesses, even to herself.

It might be as a reaction to her approach that I tend to go the other way, being hyper-aware of my body. In my case, bladder problems persuaded me to go to the doctor, and resulted in the thankfully early identification of prostate cancer (that's a different story I'll talk about later). If Mum had felt able to be more open about whatever health problems she had, might earlier identification have made a difference to her treatment? I'll never know.

In The Meantime
(A bit of further background)

So that sets the scene, but I think that before I proceed with what happened, I should explain a little more about my mum, about her background, and about the other things that had been going on during the period running up to her diagnosis.

I've said that before the dementia, Mum was strong and practical, and could deal with anything, but while that's true, that was also the *image* she liked to put out strongly to her children, over and above whatever the actual truth might be. Inside, I know she could be very insecure, worrying about me and my sister, about our family, her friends; about everything. To some extent, she no doubt felt she had to, as on top of 'generic' parenting responsibilities, my dad died from a heart attack in 1987, and she was thrown into a world where she needed to be in sole charge and raise the two of us, and be in charge and on top of everything. And for my mum, our needs and futures came first, ahead of her own. I don't have kids myself, and I'm sure that can be said of all (or most) mothers, but I think that finding yourself unexpectedly in the role of sole parent, with no-one to share that burden, makes the weight even heavier. And as Mum never wanted to show weakness either, she wouldn't seek out friendship or companionship to help support her; she'd carry the burden herself. Over the years, we even tried to encourage her when the occasional potential suitor floated around the periphery, but for Mum, we were the ones who needed the support, and, as far as I know, she never actually dated again.

She may not have mentioned it if she did toy with the idea, but the fact that she and her friends would sometimes jokingly mention admirers, always to our delight that she might find someone to make her happy, I don't think there were ever any serious contenders. I suspect she wouldn't let there be.

But even before Dad had died, I know my mum had struggled sometimes. I don't think it was ever diagnosed and we only found out later, but I think it's fairly certain Mum had been suffering from depression when we first moved to our final house at the end of the seventies. My sister and I have both had periods of counselling and anti-depressants over the years, and Mum was strong for us, but now and again she alluded to her own difficulties when we'd first moved. Not making a big deal of things, and sometimes the admissions might just have slipped out unintentionally, but she occasionally mentioned the past when discussing other subjects. One of these times occurred when I was redecorating my old bedroom in her house.

Bringing up a cuppa and observing the changes to the colour scheme, Mum mentioned casually and in passing (and not even realising what she was admitting, I suspect) that when we'd first moved to Ellesmere Port, and when my sister and I were out at school, she'd go up to my bedroom, look out over the view to the rear, and just cry; hating everything about where we'd moved to and what she was now doing (or not doing) with her life. Prior to the relocation, we'd owned a small shop in West Kirby, and

Mum had served and pretty much run the place I think, being busy and dealing with people all the time. This was before the crash of the economy that made us sell the shop in 1979. As a result of the economic traumas, she'd had to move away from her friends, and from her constant busyness, and she'd felt lost because of that. But that's a different story.

The reason I mention the anecdote is that, during this difficult period for her, she would never show us when she was upset or struggling; because you don't do that in front of your kids, particularly if you're of a certain age. In the following years, when she'd travel over to look after her own mum and dad, after my father died, she'd similarly never give any outward indication that she was struggling. Having been in that position for ourselves now, I can imagine how horrible and difficult those years and situations must have been for her. In Mum's case, she also made sure she hid that pain and distress from us, so that she could remain the strong and supportive one.

So when you consider those experiences, I guess that Mum had already undertaken decades of practice in hiding details about herself and her health. It was partly why the admission about wanting me to stay that one morning of her 'accident' had surprised me, as much as anything because she'd been saying that she needed help. And my mum didn't do that. Whenever I think back to that day, increasingly recognising it as the beginning of her loss of confidence, I imagine other issues which might already have been going on, and wonder whether this could have been a nexus point for investigating, if only I'd given it more consideration at the time. Perversely, I don't mean that if I'd pressed her,

Mum might have admitted to memory problems, as I'm certain she wouldn't have, but it actually became a distraction. In the weeks that followed, I fixated on the lack of confidence, rather than realising Mum had actually asked for help, which might have been the more important aspect of that encounter.

It's the guilt again, of course. Without us both (me and my sister) focusing on this loss of self-confidence (which mainly manifested itself in the halting of those daily trips up to the shops and going out), might we have noticed the onset of the dementia earlier? I can analyse my own thought patterns and retrospectively justify myself. The loss of confidence and not going out were connected, but I was as guilty as Mum was of ignoring the underlying root causes. In my head, if I could get her to go outside more, she'd get her confidence back, and things would go back to normal, so that was where my focus lay. I can justify why I took that approach now, but that doesn't mean I don't regret it, or feel guilty for not doing more.

Looking back, now that I'm in possession of all the facts, and analysing every decision I made as though I'd known those facts at the time, I can't yet stop the guilty feeling that I didn't manage to do anything to help Mum sooner, though hopefully I'll reach that point eventually. Logically, I know that a diagnosis of dementia wasn't even on the cards during this period, so there's no logic for this blaming myself about how I acted. But the guilt you can feel in being unable to help someone you love *is* irrational, and I have to try and remember that. To get very 'meta' about it, the best I can manage today is to keep reminding myself to not dwell on the 'what if?' But that's easier said than done, particularly if you're of an introspective and slightly OCD mentality, as I am. Even now, writing this, you can probably tell that I'm starting to go round in circles, even outdoing myself in the martyrdom stakes by starting to feel guilty about feeling guilty. It's a hard habit to break, but I think I'll leave that paragraph in as it stands, as repetitive as it might seem. It is a good reflection of my mindset. As I write this, it occurs to me that maybe I should go a little easier on myself as well, and accept some of the self-indulgent exploration of the what ifs. Guilt can be debilitating at times, but when Mum was still with us and needed looking after, I couldn't often pause to wallow in that self-indulgence for long, or even to work it through, as there was always the next day to plan and get through and new challenges ahead. Perhaps I need to do that more, to be able to let it go. On some level, that's probably why this book exists.

If you haven't been in the position of primary carer yourself, you may not realise how much recrimination and blame can prey on and haunt your mind at the time, and if this is a journey you're going through yourself, be prepared for those irrational doubts and thoughts to hang around persistently, and try to find a way to cope with them, as you're no use to anyone if you make yourself ill. I can't tell you how to do that, as everyone and every situation is different, but being aware that your experience is a common one is a good place to start. Seek out message boards online, or groups of similar carers. I didn't, as my sister and I had each other to lean on for support for practical matters, but we both might have found our own mental wellbeing much improved if we had spoken to others outside the family too. Sometimes, it's easier to share your fears with a stranger. In my case, I'm using this book (and you) to help me face up to my remaining feelings of self-recrimination, and maybe writing things down might work for you too, even if it isn't for an audience.

I try to keep the memory doctor's words to Mum in my mind as much as possible; that none of it was her fault, that these things just happen, and there's no benefit in searching for a reason. It helps me to counter the admittedly irrational fears that, in some unidentifiable way, things might be my fault too. I don't mean in a literal way, just that vague sense that there was something more I should have done, or could have done. We never really talked about those particular feelings ourselves in our family at the time, because that's 'not what we do,' but it might have helped if we had.

Talking of blame and reasons for medical problems, here's a detail I should throw into the mix, so you have a better picture of me and my mindset during this period of my life. While no medical 'explanation' was ever conclusively proven, in 2016 I spent a week in hospital after having had a minor stroke. No conclusive proof, though in my mind it was certainly a mixture of drinking, smoking and stress. I recovered pretty much completely, but had an extended period where everything from balance and eyesight to profuse sweating and scary pins and needles plagued me. My own journey here is irrelevant, but my approach to treatment and recovery was, I think, quite different.

Unlike Mum, my approach to ill-health was stoicism. I knew I was getting the medical care I needed, and that there was nothing I could do but let people look after me and heal, so I came to a kind of acceptance about my own health (and mortality). I didn't ignore it, but I accepted it, which might have been what helped me through that time mentally. But the truth of the matter is that during those weeks and months, the one worry and fear I couldn't shake was how it would affect my mum. Once I knew I was surviving, I was more worried about the effect on her than on myself. On other loved ones too, but for the purposes of the book we'll restrict this section to the concerns about my mum.

I don't know what was going on in her head when I had the stroke, but all I wanted was not to worry her, which I suppose is ironically her own fault for giving me those genes and setting that example during my upbringing. I worried how she'd cope with seeing me, travelled to visit her sooner than I was advised to so she could see I was okay, and admitted very little about how scared I'd been when it happened, or the worries about ongoing symptoms, and what it might mean for my future life and mortality. All I wanted her to see was her boy bouncing back from a minor setback, and moving on. It's exactly what she might have tried to do if the situation been reversed, and was mirrored in her own unwillingness to share her fears over her subsequent illness, not wanting to worry my sister and me about her own health.

This preceding section is all just reminder, background and setup, of course, to set the scene, so I can now go ahead and steam through some horrible, life-changing events as if they don't matter at all. I'm going to do that because this story isn't about those times; it's about Mum's dementia, but the details above are to help you get a better picture of what was going on.

Our Indestructible Mum

Even before she got properly ill, Mum hated going to hospitals and seeing doctors (and especially dentists), but a few years prior to the final illness, over the course of several months and with much loving coercion and badgering, she eventually agreed to have a lump on her neck investigated; one that we'd noticed and that seemed to be getting larger. Those early appointments don't matter here, and it turned out to be a non-cancerous growth, but she still needed to have it removed. On that horrible evening of the operation, we first went through the real worry of thinking about her mortality, and the terror of thinking our mum might die; that she wouldn't recover from the anaesthetic. The story of events leading up to that operation could also make a book in themselves, but the nuts and bolts of the danger came from the fact that Mum was a lifelong smoker, her circulation wasn't good, and she was ridiculously dehydrated due to cockups over when she'd go to the operating theatre (consequently she hadn't been allowed water for most of the day). My sister and I waited, chatting and watching TV as Mum's actual operation took place, and as her time in the 'recovery room' took longer and longer, we'd started to fret more and more. We refused the staff's repeated "suggestion" that we go home and come back to see her in the morning but, having witnessed several incidences of incompetency that day (Mum had earlier been wheeled to and back from theatre when they'd laid out the wrong instruments, then decided to switch patients rather than get the right tools) we were going nowhere until we knew she'd come through the op okay. Whatever the time might be, we weren't leaving until we saw that she was alright or, at the very least, alive! This wasn't an NHS hospital, by the way. Due to backlogs, they'd put us with the same surgeon but in a private facility, ostensibly to get their waiting lists down, I think. We'd assumed there might be better care in a private clinic. There wasn't. But I digress. Eventually Mum came back up, still insensible from the anaesthetic, not looking at all good, and although they never admitted it, I suspect bringing her round at all might have been a lot more difficult than they'd expected. But she was alive. This was the first of several times we realised how fragile life can be, and at the same time made us think that Mum must be bloody indestructible.

Mum had other health issues during her the last few years too; her digestion, hearing, eyesight, teeth, piles, swollen feet, coughing, bruising like a peach, hot water bottle burns (I was terrified about her and that bloody hot water bottle - but she was so stubborn and wouldn't accept alternatives, like microwave ones). I'm not going to detail all these illnesses, but I mention them so you understand the added challenges of the dementia. If Mum had been healthy and the dementia had progressed, it would have been difficult enough, but as with so many people when they get older, other health issues develop and accelerate too. As one of the carers, you don't just want to help with the dementia, you take responsibility for helping with all the other issues too, although the best way to deal with that, for your own sanity, is on a day by day basis, as things crop up. It's only looking back and writing this now that it really sinks in how many different aspects of Mum's health needed support, and I think it might have been too overwhelming to think about and accept all of that at the time, in anything other than the practical sense; dealing day to day, keeping meticulous records, ensuring new (and old) ailments were brought to the attention of the doctors. There was enough going on not to allow us to dwell on the big list of everything, and I'm thankful for that. I wrote earlier how Mum would never volunteer when something was wrong, and there may have been even more illnesses and problems we never got to know about, in fact there almost certainly were. It's selfish, but I'm almost glad we didn't know. And there goes the guilt again.

But, while I won't detail the litany of illnesses, there were notable major hospital scares, starting in 2017, which I should explain, as they give important context.

The first of these happened when Mum was 79, and, being superwoman, had decided to carry all the recycling boxes down our sloping drive, even though it was slippery, icy, and January. This is what we gathered later, as Mum never volunteered a clear picture of events. I think it may have been about half past ten in the morning when I got an 'innocuous text' from her while I was in work, saying that she'd had "a bit of a fall but was okay." I phoned back straight away, from work, speaking to both her and to her friend, who had been the one who finally (after much cajoling) insisted that my mother text me to let me know (yes, I'm using her more formal 'telling off' title of 'mother' deliberately). I got the basics and the gist of what the issue was, including the fact that the fall had been several hours earlier, and she was *still* bleeding from her arm. So, naturally, I panicked, though I was careful not to let that show. I jumped in a taxi (about a half hour trip), calling by phone on the way again, and letting my sister know, too.

There was a lot of blood on the kitchen floor when I arrived (and blood on the carpet in the dining room, lounge, even dotted about two foot above her height on the bathroom wall), and Mum was still sat on her stool with her friend, drinking tea, and smoking a cigarette. She'd slipped, about half eight that morning, we think, had come back inside, probably in a state of shock and, judging by the trail of blood, had sat at the table, tried to settle in the lounge, attempted to change her cardigan (hence the high blood spatters on the wall) and clean herself up and, not wanting to make a fuss, had worked on her favourite premise of "it'll all turn out alright if I just ignore it" (the most frustrating of Mum's mantras of behaviour). Her friend had arrived, I don't know what time, maybe half nine, and my mum had refused to make a fuss, or call the doctor, or let me or my sister know, and had instead sat there chatting, having cups of tea, gossiping and smoking, and all the while dripping more blood onto the tiles. Eventually, maybe having to accept things weren't improving, or to stop her friend from constantly telling her she needed to act, she'd very reluctantly texted me, and tried to downplay events when I called.

As soon as I arrived, seeing the blood and trying to appear calm, I'd wrapped her arm, grabbed a crossword book and pen, and a bottle of water, and called us a cab to A and E. Long story short, she'd broken her arm and the bone had nipped an artery, hence the continued bleeding. It might

36

even be a positive that Mum smoked, as poor circulation meant she hadn't lost as much blood as she might have. We spent hours waiting, of course, while they decided whether to operate then or not, and I had the same argument as I'd had at her last hospital visit; that if not, could she please be allowed to have some water, as she'd lost an armful of liquid already, and we'd previously had the issue of her dehydration and recovery after an operation. Mum was blindly cheerful, and we did crosswords as we waited, my sister arrived (from the other end of the country, which gives you an indication of the wait time), and we eventually settled Mum into a ward, with the op to fix her arm scheduled for the next morning.

Another slight digression here, to one of my own little pet hates. Hospital staff are wonderful, and obviously know their jobs inside-out, but are also incredibly busy people. One element they can never really know is the personality of individual patients they've never met before. As she was hooked up to a drip, I tried to explain what Mum was like to the staff nurse. If she needed the loo she would likely wait until someone happened to come past, and wave lightly like it wasn't a big deal, and apologetically explain. She wouldn't use the buzzer and bother anyone, or shout, as other patients might. If no-one came, she'd just cope with the consequences. I might be wrong about that (she was by no means a 'victim' in her mentality, though more than occasionally a martyr), but I really don't think so. Going into hospitals scared her, and she'd try to get through those times as invisibly as possible. Once she was settled, she'd be fine, and would chat to neighbours (if they spoke first); but going in, not having people she knew around her, she'd revert to her "I don't want to be any trouble" mindset. It's still a family joke, saying "I don't want to be any bother," when there's something you really want or need. Anyway, I felt I had to try and make sure they'd check on Mum occasionally, and know about her shy nature. Shifts would change and the message might not get passed on, but at least I'd tried to ensure we'd done everything that we could. I was probably a very pushy relative, and over-protective where I didn't need to be, but I know from the carers who looked after Mum later, that some would see that as her children caring so much, whereas others would just want us to go away and let them get on with their job as they saw it. And that was the sense I got in the hospital that time, that I shouldn't be trying to tell the nurse how to do her job. It would be nice if re-assuring relatives got a higher priority sometimes, as NHS staff are used to the situations which they deal with every day, but for patients and relatives it's a very scary world of new experiences.

We'd settled Mum into the ward and I stayed with her until I got kicked out, while my sister went back to the house with a vigour and determination to remove all the blood stains, knowing it would upset Mum to see them, and she did an amazing job. Perhaps we should have left some to show, so Mum would have had to accept how serious her injury, and her inaction in doing something about it, had been.

Mum had the op the next day and recovered fine from the anaesthetic (so they said), and she came home the day after that. She was still chipper and quite happy, but was obviously restricted in what she could do physically, and we spent a few weeks taking turns to look after her, as there are some things you need two hands for! We tried not to berate her too much for not calling anyone sooner, while trying to point out how serious the consequences could have been. But Mum pretended she didn't hear those arguments, or dismissed them as over-worrying. The fact is, if her friend hadn't called round, or made her finally text me, she might well have been dead already. She never let that sink in, or if she did, never showed us. Perhaps the thought scared her more than we knew, and she was even better at covering her fears than we expected. But it was also another indication of our indestructible mother.

Maybe because of this 'major scare,' we'd again been focusing on the obvious aspects of Mum's welfare, rather than worrying specifically about the mental health side. Not completely, we were already aware of, and discussing on occasion, some of the more obvious memory issues, but for a while other matters took precedence. Like our gratitude for her being still alive, and slowly getting back to full physical health.

The memory issues we'd noticed had been minor at first. Mum absolutely loved to read, for example, and would still read a wide variety of magazines and books (great when it came to finding presents) but even before her fall, there had been a slight change to that behaviour, and not just in her dwindling enthusiasm for reading. She'd swear blind she'd already read some of the books I bought for her (even though they were brand new), or when it came to watching a film, she'd sometimes be convinced she'd seen one before (despite the impossibility, as it had only just come out on DVD), or she'd swear blind that she hadn't seen a movie I knew we'd watched in recent months. And the books she had lasted much longer. She'd sometimes say that, as she was reading so many things, she couldn't remember where she was up to on one so she was going back to the beginning to start again. I suspect she'd started to forget she'd read them at all, or what had happened in the stories, and it was a struggle to keep track. I think she was so used to fibbing that it became automatic, which was where the apparent remembering things that hadn't happened (books she said she'd already read), came in. If there were too many items on her 'to read' pile (which was getting longer) or if she just didn't fancy a subject, she would claim it was a duplicate. She probably convinced herself. It was behavioural changes like these that raised questions for me and my sister, but they'd never been serious enough for us to make her see a doctor. Maybe we were scared of the answer we might get too?

Ironically, we had a fantastic time in those months after her first fall, spending more time together as a family, but it was difficult too. We both had lives and jobs and homes, and the last thing you could do was let Mum know any of them were being impacted by looking after her. She'd have been mortified, and was still "all there with her marbles," as one of her favourite sayings went. She knew she was forgetful, but for her, it was still just 'my age' and, much as with reading the books, I think she'd convinced herself that if she refused to acknowledge what was going on, problems wouldn't be real; just as she did with the fall.

I'm certain she was already having her own doubts about the future and her mental health during this period, and there were a couple of occasions when subjects related to declining health and capability were talked about openly, although always in the third person or as a hypothetical future scenario. Mum wouldn't ever want my sister or I to move back in with her if she got ill, she said. She didn't want to impact our own lives, and knew the effect it had when she and her siblings had looked after her own mum and dad, and she knew that caring wasn't a small sacrifice by any means. And, more important than that, she'd say, more than a week together and we'd all start driving one another nuts. They weren't serious, life planning conversations, not in the way they arose, but they just came up now and then. Mum may even have planned those conversations herself; she was certainly still capable of planning and worrying and fretting like that. I think it was shortly after these conversations that the "put you in a home" jokes stopped completely. It was clear from things Mum sometimes said, she would fight to stay in her own home for as long as she was physically able. I think it was in part the idea of change, the implication of what it might mean for her future, or a (totally unfounded) fear of being left without family. Over the decade before, we'd tried to persuade her to relocate to where she grew up, where she had even more family around, and we'd have visited her just as much, but to Mum, this house was "our home," and the place we came back to. And she was still 'the adult', keeping a safe place for us if we ever needed it, our home. We plan and over-worry about everything in our family, all of us.

We over-worry; that may be a slight under-statement. Tonight I keep thinking I have throat cancer. It's not hypochondria so much as a need for total control. Pre-empting illness gives you power over it. If you can pre-empt

41

and expect things, they're far less scary; that's the underlying philosophy. It was true for my actual cancer diagnosis, too. It's much easier to accept and not to panic if you've already got your worrying out in advance of the news. Not just health. Same applies to all aspects of life, like relationships and breakups; exploring the worst case scenarios allows you to avoid the surprise element of any bad news. But I digress (again).

All this background is relevant because we all pre-empt and hide in our family, and I doubt we're alone in that. I was still a child when Dad had his first heart attack, and even then, for months afterwards I worked through the possible implications of his future death; how family life might change, finances, life plans. I did it nightly, though I told no-one about this planning. When he actually died for real, a number of years later, I was far more prepared and it seemed to some I was avoiding the grief stage. But I had my plans, I was prepared, so could avoid the public grief. I was the oldest male (16), which seemed to still matter back then ("You're the man of the family now" being amongst the most popular 'condolences'). I bottled things up with everyone, even family, until one memorable evening when, in the course of an argument about nothing, I was accused of being "just like him." That broke the floodgates for me and I fled upstairs, to sob uncontrollably. Mum, of course, came up to comfort me, and I clearly remember her saying softly that they hadn't realised I was hurting so much, as I'd seemed to be fine. "Of course not," I should have said, "that was the plan, you weren't supposed to know." Why is this example important? Because it's an approach I picked up either genetically or subconsciously from Mum herself, so when she said everything was 'A' okay, when horrible things had happened, she was invariably lying and being strong, for me and for us.

Anyway, back to the events that matter. In the year following Mum's fall we started to spot even more worrying details, like cigarette burns on the carpet, in increasing numbers, where Mum had obviously dozed off, fag in hand. That was a terrifying thought, that she might burn the house down around her. I was a little more understanding of her refusal to quit. My sister has always been vehemently anti-smoking, but I'd started when I was about twelve, and had only given up in the previous year, a few months after my stroke. Mum denied they were cigarette burns from when she'd fallen asleep. They'd just mysteriously appeared on the carpet and were unrelated to her smoking. It's hard to counter that argument when there are no facts or logic to argue against. She took after my Gran, whose legendary conversation-ender of "I'm sorry, but you're wrong" indicated that a subject was closed, and it didn't matter what might be said or proved; her final word on the matter had been uttered, and that was that. Truth came second to belief.

I'll come back to the subject of fibbing several times over the coming pages ("fibbing" seems the nicest term), but it's a recurrent theme and worth highlighting again here. When I say "fibbing," what I'm talking about isn't always an intentional misdirection by a dementia sufferer, and I think is often self-deception more than anything else, but the urge for covering your tracks must quickly become a way of life when you can't remember details and specifics, and don't want anyone else to realise. I think this is what Mum had done with the cigarette burns in the carpet. She wouldn't let herself believe that was what had happened.

Anyway, as time progressed, so did our concerns over other aspects of Mum's competence and mental capabilities, such as how well she was managing her finances, and how much covering up might be involved there too. Mum was still a devotee of cash and cheques, as that's what she'd known all of her life, and she always kept meticulous records in her chequebook but in this millennium, pressures increased everywhere, first for phone banking, and then for online banking. Those can be wonderful tools, but they aren't for everyone, and I'm sure you've cursed along with me at the 'for your convenience' methods that have been introduced, which are anything but. I'm quite comfortable with technology but, dammit, I want to be able to walk into a branch and deal with a human too. But before I disappear off on a rant about modern society (I can't help it, I'm over 50), I'll drag myself back to the matter in hand.

I'd taught Mum to use a computer a few years earlier (she was already familiar with keyboards from her typing days), to send and receive an e-mail but strangely, while she had no problem at all with mobile phones, and was, in fact, quite a whizz, she was never comfortable with computers. Granted, I taught her in the days of the dial-up modem, so her written notes went to several pages, talking her through switching the computer on, waiting, to connecting to the internet, waiting, opening her e-mail program, waiting, putting in her password, waiting (you get the idea), so it wasn't much fun, and a bit like when she learned to drive, it was an objective to be able to do these things, and when she could, she lost interest. But, by the decade of the 2010s, things were much simpler, and faster, with broadband, though she still found the world of online transactions intimidating. So my sister or I would do her online banking and payments for her. I was a bit uncomfortable with this, as despite the fact I made sure she was always there and watching (or pretending to), I had no official status to make transactions on her behalf. Add to this the fact that it was frequently easier to just pay for things myself (shopping, bills etc), and being totally transparent, tell Mum and have her insist I transferred the money back to myself from her account. She kept paper lists of what she 'owed' to my sister and me, and every month we'd reckon up. While there was a paper trail, this was the other thing that made me really uncomfortable, being the one to 'give myself' money from her account.

My sister and I had a number of tentative discussions around the bogey "dementia" word and what it might mean in the future and, wanting to be as prepared as possible, this was when we looked into the idea of setting up the first Power of Attorney, for finance matters. We were lucky, actually. Our mum was always very practical, and we had relatives and acquaintances who'd recently done the Power of Attorney thing themselves, so she readily agreed we should set that up, even if it was for our own peace of mind when acting on her behalf. We made sure the forms laid around for a while to be read for several weeks, and so we didn't seem to be rushing her, but with our motto of "be prepared", it seemed sensible to get this official status put in place before we thought it might truly be necessary. That way we were both covered legally for all transactions we made, and when the time came (and we knew it would come eventually) when Mum wouldn't be capable of handling any of the money matters, we were already set up to be able to do that for her. I suspect it was a relief for Mum too, not to have to deal with one aspect of life and administration. It was a good job we did that when we did, I think. I was worried it might undermine her confidence, but she seemed happy with the general idea, even to the extent of openly admitting that we were doing it to friends and family (though of course, we always made clear that it was for logistical and audit reasons rather than due to her mental health).

So we worked through the forms with her, filled them out and left them for her to read or show to her friends or family if she wanted, and then set the date to submit the forms for the Financial Power of Attorney (POA). A very good friend of mine, who Mum had known for thirty-five years, came round to act as a witness to the document. One of the important tasks for a witness to undertake is to be the impartial individual who can confirm that they are confident that the subject of the POA is aware of what is happening and why, to make sure the person handing over financial control isn't being taken advantage of. We wanted everything to be done completely transparently and by the book. To return to the subject of fibbing, or self-deception, it's fascinating in retrospect to analyse how Mum handled this process.

There were little devices and phrases (or actions) which Mum would fall back on when there were guests present, to mask her illness and difficulties, as it's one thing close family knowing that you're having mental problems, but for as long as possible, you want to keep up the façade of normality to the outside world. I think we only became aware of some of these techniques and approaches in the latter stages, at which point it could be quite upsetting to watch, but looking back now, on this occasion she managed to tread a quite complex fine line between the truth of what we were doing, and suggestions that it had nothing to do with her memory. I think her powers of self-deception were sufficiently well-developed that Mum truly believed that some of her friends hadn't noticed her memory difficulties at all, and believed that her deceptions, sorry, her "fibbing," had been a success.

Anyway, my friend arrived and, in Mum's head and outward approach, this was just insignificant paperwork, nothing to worry about, and she was clearly determined that she wouldn't give any indication that there was an illness or weakness at play. So when the subject of the reason for my friend's visit came up, after the cups of tea were made and the biscuits cracked open, she was on sparkling form, taking the lead and explaining how she didn't want to be bothered with banking anyway, and discussing the annoyances of the inevitable shift to these online transactions, lamenting the disappearance of the chequebook, and what had been wrong with those anyway? She quite merrily discussed how she frequently had to confirm on the phone that I was speaking on her behalf when I sorted her insurance, or changed phone provider, and she really couldn't be bothered with all that, and what sort of security was it anyway? How effective is it to just hand the phone to a female voice saying, "Yes, Kit is speaking for me and is empowered to make the transactions he's raised with you." That is so true, by the way. If I really wanted to take control of the finances by phone, I could easily just get someone female to pretend they were her, and she'd have been none the wiser. I'm paraphrasing how Mum explained it, of course, but she was on form enough to make the argument that this was the reason we were applying for the POA, rather than because of any underlying health concern. Granted, on this occasion we hadn't yet had a formal diagnosis of Mum's illness, but I'd explained to her before my friend came that he already knew the full story, as he had to be in possession of the facts to be able to act as witness. When he arrived, she automatically went into "nothing is wrong" mode anyway, probably even without thinking, and I'm certain that in those moments, talking to him, that she truly believed, or had convinced herself, that we were transferring financial control almost at her own request, genuinely so that she "didn't have to bother," rather than for any other reason.

Mum's ability to seamlessly put on this convincing act that the reason for the POA was almost her idea made me wonder what else she had been performing about. Thinking back, there had been a number of earlier occasions when my queries about bills or paperwork had been met with "I'll do it later" or "Oh yes, I've sent that off," in order to make the query go away and not have to deal with further questions. Those too, I suspect now, hadn't exactly been deliberate lies, but were intended more as distractions or maybe, further self-delusion. There's always the lingering doubt (and guilt – there it is again) that I should have picked up on matters like these earlier, but no-one likes to snoop and I didn't have any reason to doubt Mum's word. In any case, what could I have actually said, if I'd suspected her answers were evasion rather than a lack of interest? I could have pressed, and asked for more detail, but that would probably have been met with even more putting off and intended distraction, or with her becoming annoyed at me, worried about getting caught out. There were occasions when Mum would be annoyed with questions, and I'm fairly sure that was the underlying reason for her getting testy. It can only ever be hypothetical now, but I wish that I'd, just once, followed up one of her vague answers around finance. It might have led to me investigating further, and realising months earlier just how much she'd been struggling, and falling behind with quite a lot of money matters. Just another one of the leftover areas of guilt.

But for now, back to the actual Power of Attorney signing. Having chatted as though nothing serious was underlying our application, my friend, who was wonderful with Mum, asked specifically if she understood what the POA meant (I was observing from a discreet distance again, in case Mum got upset by anything so I saw her nods to answer his questions, and knew exactly what she was doing). It was the mental equivalent of sticking her fingers in her ears and chanting "lalalalala". She wasn't actually engaging with what he was asking; she was doing whatever it took to make the questions go away as quickly as possible by nodding her "please don't bother me with the details" agreement.

Sorry, I was just chuckling to myself then, about something I wrote a couple of paragraphs ago, thinking back to the times when I'd made some arrangement or payment on Mum's behalf over the phone. Not only was her verbal 'approval' the most pointless and ineffectual of 'security' procedures, but as Mum's hearing wasn't exactly perfect, I usually had to stand next to her after handing over the phone, to listen in and repeat the questions from the other end, and then tell her what they wanted her to say in response. "They want to know if I have permission to make this payment, so tell them I'm acting on your behalf and with your permission." It really is a totally pointless exercise when that happens. The person at the other end must be able to hear, and know that the legal permission is just a parroting of whatever the person holding the phone is being told to say. Our approval systems for the vulnerable are so insecure, in so many ways, and the difficulty of making transactions in person just adds to that. We were very aware of that, and the POA gave me (and my sister) a little more comfort and confidence, knowing that we had the proper legal standing to act on Mum's behalf. After all, there is no telling what might be queried in the future. You hear such stories all the time, of elderly people becoming confused and paranoid, and being convinced that their family are stealing from them. While we fortunately never experienced that level of disorientation, I didn't want to be in the situation in the future where there was any doubt that I had the authority to pay the bills or deal with financial queries. Mum, of course, in her practical and deadpan way, would always take the approach, "It's yours when I'm dead anyway", trying to make light of that worry and not really comprehending that those words were hugely upsetting, and really not what we wanted anyone outside the family to hear, either. While she meant it honestly, that comment could potentially be interpreted as "I don't mind if you take my money." It's a bit like her making jokes about how we treated her, which were meant to be disarming and lighthearted, and not realising that health professionals are obliged to take a patient at their word. More on that later, but I never managed to make Mum understand that joking to a doctor "Oh yes, he locks me in the cupboard under the stairs" (or "lifts me up and puts me in the bin," which was a family in-joke) really isn't funny to an outsider, and could be a genuine cry for help in some cases, so you really can't say that to a visiting nurse or doctor. Sometimes, Mum's sense of humour was an acquired taste!

The Financial Power of Attorney came into effect in January 2018. If you're in a similar situation or think you might be at some point in the future, do it, I'd advise you to just do it as soon as you can. The process takes quite a bit of time (relatives have to be informed and people given time to object if they think it's inappropriate), and the necessity of dealing with financial affairs really is paramount. Earlier, I talked about Mum putting off questions about whether she'd sorted bills out, and when the Power finally came through, and we went through Mum's correspondence in detail, we found that there were literally dozens of uncashed out-of-date cheques, issues around the small portfolio of shares she had, out of date policies, contracts, and insurance. She'd obviously been struggling more than we knew and had at some point given up paying too much attention to everyday matters like finance completely. Her decline was more advanced than we'd realised, though day to day, a visitor still wouldn't have noticed anything different from the woman they'd always known from her conversations and demeanour. Unless you were paying deliberate attention, there wouldn't be anything amiss. But there was.

The Dementia Itself

Apologies for skipping about, but at this point it probably makes sense to jump around on the dementia timeline, and talk about the background to the crux of this journey, and the process we went through when Mum finally got diagnosed. If you're in a comparable situation yourself, or have friends going through looking after a parent or relative with cognitive impairment, it might be useful to walk through the steps of the diagnosis too.

Mum got a little vaguer about some details and subjects as 2018 progressed; just a little more forgetful, but most of the time you still wouldn't know there was a serious problem. Fortunately (in retrospect, it was quite a horrific discovery at the time), the extent of the ignored finance and correspondence pushed us to persuade Mum that she really needed to see someone to get checked out for her memory. While she tried some weak objections, the ignored paperwork and amounts of money that had gone unprocessed couldn't be ignored, even by her 'pretend nothing is wrong' approach, and with some grumbling, but beyond the stage when she could reasonably deny she was having some trouble coping, she reluctantly agreed to go with us to the doctor, who said he would refer her on for an assessment by the memory clinic, and there would be further tests for the other physical ailments we discussed, though nothing seemed to overly concern the GP. That didn't sound too scary, so we carried on as before, though as it turned out, events would overtake us before that could happen.

Mum went downhill physically in the April of that year, quite quickly and drastically. The decline was no doubt kickstarted by the combination of COPD and congestive heart failure we knew about, things we'd also pressed her to go to the doctor about, as they hadn't been formally diagnosed yet, but we knew they lurked in the background, and the continued smoking. Her circulation was getting worse, her ankles were swollen (though she denied it despite the physical evidence literally at her feet), and she'd get out of breath walking even a short distance in the supermarket. Maybe we were in desperate denial too, but when someone is still funny, laughing and joking, doing lots of puzzles, and is adamant that they feel fine, you believe everything must be okay, because that's what you want to believe.

A momentary sidebar on puzzles. Mum had always done crosswords and various word puzzles; the big one in the weekend papers, the daily ones in the Mail or the Express (don't get me started on her choice of reading matter), but for the previous year or so she'd also taken to buying books of crosswords. These were generally much easier, and smaller, but I think she did them to keep her mind active, as it's one of the things they always say in articles about memory, to do puzzles and keep your brain challenged. Up to the day before she died, Mum was doing them with us, and though some of the book ones were simple, she'd still do the ones in the paper too, and come out with obscure geographical, literary, or pop music knowledge that made you wonder, "how the hell do you know that?" Mum also loved cryptic crosswords. I know there's a knack to them, but they've always eluded me, I just can't do them. Up to the last few months, she'd cackle deliciously at my exasperation when she put in an answer to a cryptic, and had to explain to me why the buggery that was the answer. And I still didn't get it. She was a very smart woman.

But on the day of my birthday, in April 2018, I'd already realised things definitely weren't right with her, and there was no escaping that. I'd been staying overnight, as my sister and I both did quite frequently by then, and Mum had always liked to make a bit of a fuss over birthdays, though they've never been a massive deal for me personally. This particular year though, it barely seemed to register to her that it was my birthday at all. I opened cards, but while we talked about them, I don't think in the fug of her brain it really registered, what the day was. And later, she called me through to her bedroom, a bit worried as she'd caught her leg on something and it was bleeding. It was bleeding quite a lot. Her legs were quite swollen, and her skin was very thin anyway, but whatever she'd caught it on had caused a cut that just refused to stop bleeding. I bandaged it and we called the doctor. I won't go into extended detail but it was a nasty, pernicious cut, and it needed the dressings changed every few days at Outpatients. We arranged to see the Practice Nurse at the doctors, as well (it was so hard to actually see a doctor without seeing a triage nurse first at her surgery). The nurse was quite officious, and clearly busy, but didn't really listen as I tried to raise wider issues, and discuss the other health problems that we knew existed. She wouldn't prescribe anything without a barrage of tests, which Mum was dead against, and we went through the usual performance of Mum being asked what was wrong, her laughing nervously and saying, "nothing really," and the nurse not listening to what I described, as the patient wasn't saying it herself. It was so frustrating, for us all probably.

Matters didn't improve over the next couple of weeks. I called the doctor (or Duty Prescribing Nurse) out to the house a couple of times, claiming an 'emergency,' as that seemed to be the only way to get someone to actually come and see Mum in person, rather than guess what to do from the other end of a phone, and Mum was in no fit state to leave the house most of the time.

On the 26th of April, my sister was 'on duty' and looking after Mum, and she phoned me while I was at work, really concerned. We'd been worried for a day or two about how Mum was acting and how unwell she seemed, but things were clearly worse that day, and my sister had been fobbed off when she tried to get the doctor back out. I put in my "Mr Angry" eyes and phoned with the "I won't accept a refusal; someone needs to come out now" script, and got in a cab to come over too. Mum was laid back in her recliner chair when I arrived, cup of tea untouched (unheard of, and a definite sign that there was a genuine problem), 'resting her eyes,' not really taking in the fact I was present at all. The doctor came after lunch, took her pulse and blood pressure, and roused Mum enough to talk to her and ask if she knew what was going on, and told her that she was a grey colour, and needed to let us take her to hospital. She refused. He (thankfully) firmly pointed out if we couldn't call an ambulance now, we'd be calling an emergency one within 24 hours. With resentful looks at us, and complaints that she felt like "she was being hijacked," and maybe with the adrenaline kicking in, she seemed to be more herself. With a quite typical stubbornness and contrariness, she refused to leave with the ambulancemen until she'd had a cigarette and finished it. We could tell she was scared stiff. She wasn't the only one. This didn't seem like a mild illness.

They put Mum in a wheelchair and I went with her in the ambulance while my sister brought the car, and once there, on the ward, Mum perked up (of course, awkward sod!). They did a number of tests and we all did some crosswords together, our helpful distraction and a calming mechanism for everyone. It's a blur now exactly how it happened, but within a couple of hours Mum had stopped responding to the oxygen and she was moved into the emergency area. I don't know how long we were in there, but the reactions around us indicated that this wasn't just precautionary, and the faces and kind smiles suggested that this might possibly be the end of her life. How we got there from crosswords and chatting a couple of hours earlier, I have no idea. Everything was a blur, and I don't think I was even that scared outwardly. It seemed too abstract and unreal for that, and maybe I was in denial too, but it was horrific.

And then it wasn't just vague indications. We were asked about a DNR, a "Do Not Resuscitate" notice. As the staff explained, the seriousness sank in even more. The DNR is often a kindness, not a negative. To resuscitate in ICU, they have to be violent, and it isn't pretty. It really is a last resort. More details followed. While there would only be a remote chance an attempt at resuscitation would work anyway, it would certainly be painful, excruciating in fact, and would damage her body, so that even if she beat all the odds and recovered, the necessary harm done might leave her permanently incapacitated. It might be the case that, if we loved her, the greatest kindness would be to avoid putting her through that. We very reluctantly agreed for the DNR to be signed. I hope you never find yourself in that situation, I really do. It seems such a small thing, to agree to sign a piece of paper, but the meaning is life-changing. Which is probably the most inappropriate description I could use. Every view we got from the different doctors was the same; if you want to avoid seeing your mum in pain, agree to this, as it's almost certain she wouldn't survive the experience anyway and, if she did, it would just mean further pain and distress for her, and in all likelihood, would just be a very slight delay. I think there was a kind of numbness as we agreed, shock and disbelief at what was happening still clouding everything. It didn't seem real.

You don't need to know exactly what it was like for us as that day steamrolled on and, suffice to say, it was one of the worst evenings we'd ever had. But miraculously, and God knows how, our indestructible mother survived that night and came through again, though not without immense personal cost.

What followed were weeks on the ward, oxygen, emphysema, a lesion on her pancreas, infections. We'd need to make significant changes all round for her to be able to come back to her home. We'd have to make the arrangements we needed to, changes to the house (rails, key safe, alarms, various movement aids), would have six weeks of the re-ablement team of carers visiting four times a day to look after her, and a new medicine regimen. There was so much to plan and do, but keeping busy probably saved our sanities. And of course, at the centre of it all, there was a very scared old lady.

Occupational Health were next on our list to speak to, to look at changes to the house that might be needed, most of which would be free. This was obviously in order to totally preclude any debate within families over 'whether we actually need something and if money should be spent on infrastructure rather than care.' The experts decide what is needed, and make the necessary arrangements to put support features in place. It was wonderful of them, and anything that takes a decision away from the unqualified carer is very welcome when there is so much else going on, and when you need to spend all your time with the patient.

We made various other changes to the physical accessibility and layout of the house, to break routines, and hopefully make things easier for Mum to adjust. For example, Mum obviously wouldn't be smoking ever again, but her previous routine had her with her ciggies and paper at the kitchen table. So we turned the table to face the other way round. A minor change, but hopefully enough of a subtle alteration that the familiar routine would be broken subconsciously (my sister's idea). We never told Mum why we'd done that, but it seemed to work. There was a slight repositioning of her chair and a change to replace the gas fire with an electric one (she was having trouble manipulating the knob to light it, and the possibility of gas just leaking out haunted us). Mum didn't like it at first; she never liked change at the best of times. But accepted the necessity, and I think knew, that the alterations we were making would increase her chances of staying in her own home, so she went along with them. In addition to the changes we made, she'd need a lot of additional help, for a while at least.

This is where I'll jump forward to pick up the dementia angle of the story again, from when Mum got home from hospital, but not at all herself. I'll return to the story of her physical care later in a subsequent chapter. But in terms of mental acuity, when she was discharged, it seemed that we might be 'spared' Mum's gradual descent into the dementia we knew was there, only to have that fear replaced with the horror that "our Mum," as we knew her, might have already mentally left the building, as it were. It wasn't the same woman who came home, and although she seemed outwardly okay during the daytime, if quieter and more reserved, we knew it was time to accelerate the plans that had been discussed earlier. We knew that tough times lay ahead, and that having to make some difficult decisions would upset her as well as confuse her so, in May 2019, with Mum's agreement, we applied for the Health Power of Attorney.

My friend did the honours as witness again, and Mum was bright and perky once more, confirming that she wanted to go ahead with this PoA too. I can't remember the exact words of our discussions, but I know the issue of her memory and illness was vocalised very explicitly this time, and I'm fairly sure we used the term "dementia" openly, but Mum's approach was still, in exactly the same way, to selectively not hear those terms, I think. She'd carry on the conversation, putting on the front of being her old self, while saying she thought this was for the best, and that it saved her having to deal with complicated forms, which was her justification for wanting to proceed, rather than admitting to her dementia. I left them alone for a few minutes each time the witnessing occurred, knowing my friend could be trusted, but wanting him to have the chance to ask anything he needed to ask, free of my observation or influence. I think it's vital to have a witness not just to sign the form, but to actively engage and be totally transparent about the process; not least of all to try and wheedle out if Mum had any doubts herself that she might not be willing to tell us about. Mum was happy and perky throughout the process and seemed perfectly content with the forms being set up.

It was only at this relatively later stage, seeing Mum "on form" despite the problems we now knew she was having, that I started to consider just how often she might be "performing" for me and my sister too, and how much we could really trust her word about anything; about her health, how she might genuinely be feeling at any given point, or any discomfort she might be in. It became one of the very real worries we constantly had in the last months, knowing full well that Mum would put on a front, self-deception or otherwise, rather than ever complain or admit anything was wrong. There's a crawling discomfort when you have to admit that you can't trust what a parent says to you and, at least for me, it felt like it was me in the wrong for having that distrust. It was a particular concern when Mum had visits from the external care company in the last months. If anything happened to upset her, even if she remembered by the time she spoke to us, Mum would never likely volunteer details of any problems, and would pretend everything was fine. We had our own little ways of trying to wheedle details out of her at that stage. It's partly where the title of this book comes from.

When we were young, Mum used to frequently ask "did anything interesting happen at school today," which I later discovered was a suggestion from a book on parenting. I remember noticing her starting to ask this on a regular basis soon after I began having panic attacks at Junior School (as we called it in those days), and the theory is apparently that casual discussion is more likely to prompt someone to reveal unusual or upsetting occurrences, without feeling as though they're being interrogated. If you talk about what happens every day, you're more likely to reveal events which might have hurt or upset you. So the plan in that case was to see if anything at school was triggering the panic attacks, I presume. There wasn't, they were just panic attacks and the sudden daily questions were so blatant I figured that out and wouldn't have said anyway. But when Mum deteriorated, we would ask daily (or every time we called), "has the lady been yet?" meaning the scheduled care visit. As well as checking up on the company, it was a good way to gauge what Mum remembered each day; if it was a good day and she could remember the name of the carer and what they'd said, or whether it would just be a generic "yes" or "no," which usually meant she wasn't certain if she'd even had a visit. There are so many associated symptoms as dementia progresses too, that this indication of how she answered a regular, bland query could be a useful pointer to confusion, frustration and mood, as well as forgetfulness. On occasion she'd snap back that we didn't need to ask that question every day, which told us that she remembered the routine, knew what we were trying to find out, and was as annoyed at the dementia, or at herself, as she was with us. Oddly, that might well indicate that she was having one of her better days, at least in terms of recall and self-confidence.

John Stiles (son of footballer Nobby) was on TV the other day, talking about his dad's dementia and how people's perceptions of it as a disease are varied. Particularly if it's something like "Mixed Dementia" (as it was with Mum), which doesn't have a recognisable label like "Parkinson's" or "Alzheimer's," so seems strangely lesser. His point was that dementia isn't inevitable, isn't just old age or confusion; it's actually brain damage. If viewed in that way, it might be looked at quite differently by society. Watching the interview, I couldn't decide whether I found that description scarier or more comforting than simply "dementia." It did make me realise though, that after Mum's last stay in hospital, where lack of oxygen was such a significant issue and had put her in the emergency room, that an acceleration or increase in brain damage, and of the outward signs of dementia, makes complete logical (if not emotional) sense. There was no pretending it could be anything other.

The Diagnosis

So now I'll jump forward to the actual diagnosis of dementia, so you can understand what we went through to inform our planning for Mum's care after her hospital visit. It wasn't just about her physical frailty; whatever we put in place had to be the best way to support Mum's mental needs as well.

This isn't actually much of a jump in the timeline. As I mentioned, we'd visited the doctor at the beginning of the year to get a referral to the memory specialists, but as flawed as NHS systems often are, the referral (which should have happened on April 17th) never went through, so it was actually several months later, after Mum's hospital stay and her near-death experience, and after we'd had to cope with her gradual recovery, that we finally got the process of formal assessment moving. When that appointment finally arrived, it started with a home visit from the specialist memory team. This was an initial assessment visit, where a professional from the memory clinic came out to do the first evaluation of Mum's mental state and acuity. We tried to make this into a bit of a game, to make the experience easier and less intimidating for the old lady. It was nerve-wracking for all of us I think, Mum, my sister and me, and while we took it very seriously, making sure we had a less pressurised attitude to the appointment seemed the most sensible and stress-reducing approach.

As you might expect, to begin there were a number of broad questions to see if Mum was aware of world events, dates, and what was taking place in the news, to gauge the more obvious signs of confusion or dementia. She 'passed' with flying colours. So far, so good. Next, there were a number of little practical tests, though thankfully nothing too taxing or daunting. They might give a name and address, for example, and several times throughout the course of the visit, they'd go back to those details and ask again, to find out how well the information had been retained. It was a bit like a gameshow in some respects and, helpfully, Mum did like her gameshows and quizzes, so it didn't feel too 'medical,' or too much like an exam. She was nervous, naturally, and as we anticipated, her recall wasn't exactly perfect. I sat alongside to re-assure where I could, while fighting back my natural urge to intervene and help (and to answer on her behalf).

For weeks after this visit, my sister and I carried on with an intermittent 'testing' of Mum's ongoing recall of the name and address she'd been given to memorise during the assessment, relieved that some of the information seemed to have stuck. That re-assured Mum too, knowing she was able to retain information longer term, and that we knew she could do that. When we did ask if she remembered the address, it was done in the form of the casual 'gameshow' approach (win a prize if you remember the exact details), so it seemed more like a game we were playing than a further examination, and she took this in good sport. As we'd discover later, repetition and familiarity can be re-assuring and welcoming to sufferers of mental disorders, so we may have inadvertently made the whole experience more palatable by repeatedly asking in that way. One side effect was that the address she'd had to remember was burned into my own memory for several months too. I still remember now that it was Cherry Tree Lane, and could probably remember the whole thing if I put my mind to it. To be frank though, it isn't information that would bring me any pleasure, and when I've considered it, even brings an uncomfortable sensation I might be testing my own memory abilities by thinking I should retain that meaningless bloody address.

Anyway, it was a very nice and understanding lady who'd visited to do this assessment, and one thing I will say, over the course of the final three years, is that I personally came to trust the approach and collaborative knowledge of many medical professionals less. But the specialists around memory... I came to trust them far more. Understandable, I'm sure, as they have the skills and experience to know how to deal with sufferers of mental degeneration, while some nurses and general practitioners don't always have the time or intuition to realise how carefully and slowly you occasionally have to tread, in order to get useful answers for diagnoses. This lady was wonderful with Mum. When a patient doesn't like admitting that they're ill at all, and are often also naturally disposed towards minimising concern ("I don't want to be any bother" – the semi-joking catchphrase in our family), it's frequently difficult to get the correct information for diagnoses, because sufferers like Mum don't want to admit and share the details of their specific problems. Understandably in the main, medical staff always want to hear direct from the patient (rather than from the relative or carer) just in case there is coercion or covering up/maltreatment involved. But if you combine someone who is already reticent to admit they have any issues, with a new set of genuine problems in remembering details and information, then the search for diagnostic evidence gets very complex. This is where the general medical staff aren't always equipped or experienced enough to find answers.

One example of this kind of issue which springs to mind had arisen a few years earlier when, after much cajoling, Mum had finally agreed to go and see her doctor (not 'her doctor' of course, as the surgery had changed to the current, and more 'efficient', model of seeing whoever was on duty that day) about an unrelated but ongoing medical problem. As the doctor on duty didn't know Mum personally, they had no background knowledge or relationship with her, to make the encounter more productive, and he had no context for knowing her personality or shyness. When we got into the consulting room, Mum immediately reverted to type, and on being asked what the matter was, just smiled apologetically, saying "nothing really," that she was fine, and didn't know why we were bothering the busy doctor. Mum really didn't want to be seen to complain, and to be fair, it must have been exceedingly difficult for the doctor to know how to treat a patient who comes in and then denies that there's anything wrong with them. That was why my sister or me always accompanied Mum to medical appointments; not only to support, but in order to cajole and provide the details she wouldn't volunteer herself, stuck in her mental approach of 'don't admit there's an issue and it will go away on its own, eventually.'

But I digress. With memory specialists, they know from repeated experience that, for the genuine facts, you usually need to talk to the patient's relatives or carers as well as the individual, and these memory professionals are pretty astute at picking up what familial relationships really are. A little sidebar here, as it just occurred to me to mention it, is about the comments we'd sometimes receive throughout the last few years, and which surprised me greatly; the number of times we were told by medical and mental health specialists how lovely it was to deal with a family so invested and involved in every aspect of Mum's care. I'm sure they equally thought we were pains in the arse and interfering at times, but the consistent message was how nice it was to see family wanting to be so involved and making sure every detail of Mum's support was as good as it could be. I'm not blowing our own trumpets; to some extent, our circumstances probably created a particular closeness. My dad died when I was sixteen, and Mum raised us both on her own after that, never re-marrying or even being properly involved in any relationship. We were very close, and it can't have been easy being my mum at times. I had my own issues around depression and anxiety, mixed fortunes in life, but she was always there. Neither my sister nor me were married, or had kids, so Mum was always still the family we returned to; at Christmas-time, or at times of trouble. We were a close family in those ways, so it was only natural that, when it became time for us to take the responsibility route, we took a very detailed approach to every aspect of our mum's care. I understand others will have far more calls on their time than we did, and their own families to put first, but concerning matters like the specific details of a care package, or making sure that Mum was aware and supported at every stage of the process, we wanted and needed to do everything that we humanly could. I don't understand how people wouldn't want to do that, but it seems, from the comments we received, that many people inexplicably don't. I'm not judging, because every situation and family bond is different, I know, but if you take the responsibility for care, I just don't understand how you wouldn't then do that to the best of your ability. I'm digressing. Sorry.

Anyway, during the memory assessment itself, I'd tried to stay out of the questions and answers as much as I could, but had made sure I was about and in easy reach, in case Mum got upset, and also so that I was available to flag where Mum might be volunteering less than the total truth.

Fortunately, Mum was on good form and was fine with the whole assessment and testing process on the day, didn't get too flustered, and we all had a nice chat afterwards. By this stage in the dementia journey, Mum was consciously aware that she was undeniably having memory problems, and though we still avoided actual terms like "dementia" where we could, so she wouldn't panic (substituting terms like "forgetfulness," "things slipping her mind" etc), I'm sure that she knew deep down what the real situation was. I suspect it was actually a relief to her, to have the option of trying to keep hiding the problems taken away. It must have been so exhausting for her to try and hide what was happening to her all of the time.

Anyway, it was fairly obvious to the lovely lady who came out for the initial mental competence assessment, that there were more issues here than simple ageing, and we subsequently got referred on to the next stage of diagnosis, and before too long we had an appointment at the Memory Clinic itself, in a place called Cherry Orchard House (November 2018, 11am, if you care about such details). There were no Cherry Trees or Orchards in the immediate vicinity, so maybe it was named after the colour of the fire engines at the station next door, or the trees they cut down to clear the land for the buildings. I'm guessing it was where the Cherry Tree Lane of the memory assessment came from too. Bloody, memorable, address.

I think I was almost more nervous than Mum about this next, actual appointment, with a real doctor, but having said that, it was very clear that she didn't want to go into the building at all either, and would use any method she could in order to delay or avoid the meeting, where she knew she'd have to confront and talk about her mental health quite openly. There was no turning back from that point. Mum was quite slow walking from the car to the door, reminding me a little of the child who takes the approach that delaying the inevitable might somehow make it not happen, but I made no comment, walked equally slowly, smiling and making distracting comments, and we finally got there and sat down, and further distracted ourselves with crosswords as we waited (if it was possible, crosswords should sponsor me for praising them so much). As usual, the puzzles helped to calm nerves and move concentration away from the appointment to come.

We had another minor challenge here, one which might not be unfamiliar, and which had the potential to be quite awkward. The doctor, who was very pleasant and friendly, had a fairly thick accent, and Mum wasn't the best at understanding strong accents, of any type. I can't recall where her accent was from, as I'm absolutely rubbish at identifying them myself, but if I had to guess I'd say it was of South Asian origin. It's quite strange, as one of Mum's closest friends has quite a strong Thai accent, and she had no problem at all with understanding her, so it might be more accurate to say that Mum had difficulty understanding some new accents in people she didn't know, and particularly in stressful situations. Add to this the fact that we're talking about a woman ingrained with politeness, finding the idea of someone realising she couldn't understand their words to be slightly mortifying.

Here, we actually benefited, I think, from Mum's new-found ability to "fake understanding," as my sister and I had started to become adept at spotting her 'tells.' I could frequently identify when Mum hadn't understood what was being said to her during a complicated or emotional conversation. In this case I don't necessarily mean the technicalities of what was being explained; I mean I could easily sense the nods and bland smiles that meant she was trying to bluff her way through not following details because of the accent. That gave me the opportunity to prompt a little, repeating questions in a more familiar voice which put Mum at ease, and maybe phrasing questions slightly differently to make answering more straightforward. It wasn't just the accent issue, of course Mum also didn't always understand exactly what was being asked of her, and would try to revert to bland nods and nervous laughter as a matter of course.

The doctor would sometimes clearly speak directly to my mum without my interpretation (ok, read "interruption"), but that risked Mum coming back with generic answers about being fine, and there being nothing amiss, partly because of her reticent nature, but also because she hadn't understood what she'd been asked. It's a delicate balancing act as a carer or family member at the appointment; needing to get the history across accurately but also, where possible, having Mum tell those facts for herself. We muddled through it, with a mixture of me holding my tongue while the initial questions were asked and unhelpful answers given, or an awkward silence where Mum wasn't able to guess at the question, at which point I'd pipe up and rephrase the question myself, and try and persuade and nudge towards the truth, but getting Mum to be the one to say or admit it. It worked, well enough, anyway.

We discussed family health history, and I added a few extra prompts to make sure anything relevant was disclosed; illness in other relatives, previous health difficulties, specific occasions of memory loss, and presenting the reason for the assessment being that my sister and me were a bit concerned, blaming ourselves for the appointment, trying to take the onus off Mum so she didn't feel 'got at.' My contributions at this point also gave me the opportunity to add in details about how Mum would sometimes seem, and be, stressed by appointments and tasks she didn't like doing, and I added descriptions of the panicky moments she sometimes had, when situations seemed overwhelming, and Mum's subsequent tendency to internalise and wind herself up further as a result. I told the doctor that we worried this might be related to the mental condition, in addition to the "forgetting" parts. Mum would never have volunteered that information herself, but I wanted the doctor to have the full picture, including all the potential symptoms we'd observed. Nothing seemed to surprise her. Like I say, memory specialists see a lot, and I think are very familiar with reticent, scared, or quiet patients, like Mum.

After a while, the doctor asked if Mum wanted to hear the initial diagnosis herself, based on the earlier tests and our discussions, and I took her hand as she faked a happy smile and answered a very shaky "yes" (meaning "not really, no, I can't think of anything I'd like less"). The doctor was wonderful with her, and asked Mum what she herself thought the problems might be. Mum said, "old age," with a little attempt at a distraction laugh. But when asked in a bit more detail what that might mean, Mum admitted that she didn't really know (I think meaning that she did know exactly, but didn't want to say the words out loud, as saying them aloud might make this real). I was jotting notes as we went, for my own reference as much as for Mum's, as these situations are so overwhelming for everyone, it's easy to miss phrases or important suggestions. That's why I know all these details now, a couple of years on. We still have the notes. If you end up in similar assessments, I'd recommend always taking notes as you go. It's amazing the minute details that prove invaluable.

The doctor asked me what my sister and me thought the diagnosis might be, and I said that we'd discussed it, and we assumed we were talking about some form of dementia. It was awkward using that word in front of Mum, as we still tended to use euphemisms, but you reach a point when details have to be addressed head on, and Mum needed to hear and accept the actual words.

The doctor confirmed that we were right, gave us lots of booklets to read, and talked slowly and thoroughly through what dementia meant in reality, as opposed to what we (and you) might have heard or read elsewhere. As I'd expected, Mum pretty much zoned out during this part of the discussion, nodding occasionally, but clearly having reached the point where the best way to cope was to pretend nothing of import was being said. She let me take in the details, knowing we'd go through it all when we got home, when she was more comfortable.

To be able to accurately diagnose, and to provide any of the types of medication that might help, the doctor suggested a scan was needed, to try and identify the illness behind the dementia; Alzheimer's, for example. Despite the fact that Mum's concentration had deliberately wandered off to a happy place to avoid dealing with a reality she didn't like (mentally watching squirrels perhaps), a part of her brain was clearly still alert and paying attention, as the word "scan" was barely out of the doctor's mouth before she stated that she was unequivocally not having an MRI. At various times, different specific ideas became the bogey term, and on this day, it was MRI. Mum had one once before and was scared of being stuck in the small tube (which I quite understand; I absolutely hate the bloody things, having had over half a dozen myself for various complaints and illnesses). After joint cajoling by me and the doctor, she very reluctantly agreed to have a CT scan instead. It was one of those strangely wonderful moments, when having achieved her "victory" of not having to have an MRI, Mum actually relaxed a fraction. She had a small piece of control back, and as with other experiences, I don't think there's anything better for someone going through the no-doubt overwhelming and undermining experience of creeping dementia, than feeling you have control over something, however small. As a result of this 'victory' on her part, the rest of the consultation went even better, with Mum's biggest fear (I think she'd visualised or compartmentalised the dementia as an MRI, which she'd now avoided) being successfully sidestepped, so that option was now in the past and able to be ignored. Mum even seemed happier discussing some of the other more awkward terminology.

The scan itself was to be scheduled at the local hospital, probably within three months, and the doctor talked about the two types of medication that might likely help and would be fine to administer as Mum "had no vascular problems." To return to my receding lack of confidence in general practice, I quickly jumped in and detailed the congestive heart failure which Mum suffered from (although I did make a slight prat of myself by calling it "congenital heart failure" by mistake, and asking the doctor "are you sure?" when she corrected me). The heart condition surprised the doctor, and she told us that this fact could have significant implications for the safety of the medication she'd intended to give. There was nothing in Mum's notes from the GP about the congestive heart failure, and the doctor said she would contact the surgery. This is a perfect example of why it was imperative that one of us was there for the appointment. Aside from the fact that Mum wouldn't have volunteered that information herself even if she'd remembered it, I was learning not to trust that communication between health agencies happened as it should. And this was a potentially life-threatening detail when it came to the medication.

When we got back home from Cherry Orchard House, I e-mailed the memory specialist's secretary with a transcript of my sister's most recent conversation with Mum's GP, so that she could more easily track the pertinent place in her notes where the diagnosis around the vascular issues should be. I can't stress enough the importance of keeping detailed notes at every stage of this long and complicated process. You never know when the next health professional might need to know some pertinent fact, date, or diagnosis. One lesson ingrained in me from that point; don't assume that the information a specialist has received is complete or accurate. My sister created a folder for all these things; financial, medical, legal; so we had everything at hand when we needed it.

After e-mailing, I rewrote my notes from the consultation, neatly, legibly and in order (something we were doing every time we had an appointment by now), and read them through with Mum in a less pressurised situation, with a cuppa, answering her questions, letting her see I was hiding nothing from her, making sure she knew what had been said and agreed, and leaving the notes themselves for her to read whenever she wanted. A copy would be scanned into our own 'medical file' and e-mailed to my sister later that day. During this whole journey, every step is into the unknown, and I had no idea how Mum might react, how much she'd taken in, or what questions there might be but it seemed, on the surface at least, that all was fine this time. She actually asked some questions too, so she wasn't ignoring the entire process, and that was a relief.

Jump forward a few weeks and the CT scan passed, again surprisingly, without incident. Our follow-up with the memory doctor for the results was due in the February, and as Mum wasn't up to leaving the house on the intended date, we had a home visit instead, this time with my sister present (we took turns attending these appointments where we could).

The doctor talked to Mum about her mood, about how she felt, and, as usual, confronted with someone she didn't really know (or possibly didn't remember), Mum was very upbeat about everything that was raised or discussed. She was fine, everything was fine, it was all a bit of a fuss over nothing really, wasn't it? Of course, it wasn't. At this appointment, my sister mentioned the other curious symptom which had started recently. Mum had a hiatus hernia when she was a little younger, but something which could have been related to that had started happening recently, or rather not happening, with her digestion. Particularly with main meals, Mum frequently wouldn't be able to eat what was on her plate and would feel physically sick, and quite often be, not exactly sick, but bring up lots of phlegm. Not a pleasant experience, upsetting for us seeing it, so obviously hugely upsetting for Mum herself; not knowing why this was happening, but becoming anxious at the very thought of eating, which in turn could naturally increase the frequency of the digestive issues.

We'd wondered whether the whole thing might be anxiety-related, as no physical explanations could be found (and Gaviscon was already a part of the daily routine), but this symptom didn't seem to have any direct relevance to the dementia. Nothing much could be done about it by the memory specialist of course, she worked in a different field; however, she did suggest we maybe try smaller, less intimidating portions (although they were frequently children's' meals already), and encourage Mum to eat less but more often. It was so nice to have someone actually listen and suggest solutions rather than just pass symptoms off in the vain hope a random 'test' might show the solution. It gave us something to attempt, and the frustration of our journey so far was that there was so little we could actually 'do,' so we received the suggestion gratefully.

This digestive problem was a worry for us beyond the discomfort of the vomiting itself. To take events just slightly out of order here, by this stage we had the carers coming to visit four times a day (next chapter) and the result of these bouts of sickness was that Mum was starting to avoid eating where she could, which was a big concern. It started to become a regular occurrence that when teatime carer called, she would find the plate of sandwiches that had been left at lunchtime ("because I'm not hungry yet"), with the food still untouched. Cheese, crackers and biscuits were the only welcomed food which, let's face it, aren't the healthiest or most digestible of foods themselves, and weren't going to help her get the vitamins and nutrients she needed. But the fact Mum that seemed okay eating these unhealthy foodstuffs with no problems backed up our suspicion that this symptom must be, at least in part, psychological. There may have been something genetic at play too. As a child, when I first started to suffer from panic attacks, the nature of these attacks often came in the form of feeling (though rarely being) sick. Perhaps there was, and is, something in our genes that means this is how our bodies react to worry or anxiety. Combine that with a lifetime as a smoker, chest problems and a build-up of phlegm, and we could have had a combination of causes for Mum.

Our 'psychological cause' suspicions were further supported by the fact that this sickness wasn't consistent and didn't always occur. Sometimes Mum could tuck into full meals, and even have seconds, with no problems, and we gradually discovered that one way to encourage this seemed to be to distract her from thinking about the fact that she was eating. Mealtimes when my sister and I were there would be full of talk and conversation, and with a small crosswords book or daily Countdown puzzle on the table to be attempted as we ate (and the sick bowl, just in case, discretely out of sight under the table). It helped some of the time. There are so many tips and tricks that you discover, to help deal with the various aspects of illness; Some you can explain or justify, others just seem to help for no identifiable reason, but this method of 'distraction' became increasingly useful. And this, we could surmise, had a logic to it. If there is an element of anxiety associated with illness, and there often is with dementia, taking someone's attention away, to an essentially 'safe space' of a puzzle or crossword, means the sufferer isn't dwelling on or obsessing over what might happen next.

But I'm going off piste again. This was just the first time we'd raised the specific problems with digestion directly with a medical professional who seemed to take an interest, and had some ideas about what we might try to help. She seemed to care far more than the GP did, even though it was outside her direct sphere and remit.

The home visit by the memory doctor also delivered the results of Mum's tests and CT, and the summary of the brain scan indicated what she called age-related shrinkage, with Mum's blood vessels stiff and less pliable, so poor blood supply was deemed the most likely reason for some of the memory issues. This fitted with a history of smoking, congestive heart failure and COPD. There were no indications of stroke or Alzheimer's-related problems. We learned that diagnoses in this field are rarely of one 'pure category,' so Mum's illness would be defined as 'mixed dementia,' though it was presumed to be primarily vascular driven. None of this came as a huge surprise, though for me at least, there was a slight sense of perverse disappointment. I know we're all too obsessed with labels these days, but having a defined and 'named' type of dementia would in some ways have been easier, for me at least. I wrote earlier about feeling helpless and unable to take identifiable steps to assist, and if it had been Alzheimer's or Parkinson's, at least we might have been able to research specifics, or join online message groups. Not that either of us is particularly sociable, but even lurking and reading, without taking part, would have been something for us to do. I know that helped me later when it came to dealing with my own cancer.

In terms of treatment, we were told that memory medications weren't really effective in this instance (and would be more applicable to Alzheimer's-related conditions), so the doctor wasn't going to be prescribing any tablets. Those were the facts.

Next, the doctor reminded Mum that none of this was her fault, and was just the way brains are, with some people more susceptible than others as they get older. But I don't think that really went in. Again, now that we were in a serious discussion, Mum's concentration was probably somewhere else, anywhere else, so she didn't have to try and understand or cope, knowing we'd be noting everything down so she didn't need to focus if she didn't want to. And she definitely didn't want to.

Social and mental activities were the best therapy that existed for this type of dementia, and we talked about Mum not reading books as much as she used to in the last couple of years. From a medical standpoint, we were told, someone gets the same benefits from re-reading the same things over as trying something new, so perhaps we could encourage her to start reading again; short, non-intimidating reading materials. It didn't matter if she'd read books or magazines before. We liked that. It was something else we could do, something practical, and those things were few and far between.

Now that a diagnosis had been made, the doctor suggested that practical advice and help could also be sought from Admiral Nurses or the Alzheimer's Society (even though the diagnosis was 'mixed dementia' rather than actual Alzheimer's). We were told that via social services, there are also support groups or the option of a 'befriender' as a contact, someone who might take Mum out/ chat to her regularly, etc. We quickly discounted that on practical terms. Mum could be the life and soul of a conversation, but being outgoing and meeting new people wasn't really her wheelhouse even before all this, so suggesting she make friends with a stranger seemed unlikely to work and, to be frank, felt a bit patronising. She still had her own friends around, after all.

The final outcome of the visit though, disappointingly for us as the memory doctor had been fantastic, was that Mum would be signed back to her GP because there was nothing else the specialist could really do which Admiral Nurses (et al) couldn't. But the memory doctor told us that Mum could be referred back again by the GP if needed. Mum's Sertraline could easily be upped to help her mood if necessary, but this would be via the GP, and Mum's reactions and conversation during the visit suggested to the doctor that it didn't seem necessary at that time, as there weren't any real signs of serious depression.

This storytelling of mine probably seems quite disjointed to you. Being honest, that's partly by my own design, as frustrating as it might be for you. Frustration is the key overriding emotion for the carers and relatives (and for the patient) as all this is going on, and if you want to understand what it was like for us, that's also the description. Frustrated, and scared, and feeling lost. You think a route is going to lead to a solution, but new problems come out of left field, improvements one day are gone the next, and vice versa. The memory doctor had been an amazing help; in the diagnosis, in supporting us, in persuading Mum this was real, but now that part was done, it was on to the challenges of everyday life. And throughout this period, we'd also been dealing with the increasing physical challenges for Mum. So, to jump back a year, to the point when she'd first been discharged from hospital after the near fatal consequences of her admission in April 2018...

Carers and Caring

For a number of weeks, after a spell in in hospital like Mum had, the NHS provides a team of carers for free, to visit and look after the discharged patient, to help them adjust to the new reality of the loss of physical abilities, to a new routine, and to help the family understand just what will be needed for the future. The "re-ablement" team was amazing, and I can't praise them highly enough.

Initially, even though the carers from the team visited four times a day to help Mum with getting up, meals, pills, getting ready for bed, etc, my sister and I also stayed every night; to be there and do whatever we could, and to make the situation as normal as we could for her. It also helped us to see exactly what might be required, going forwards. It was a strange time for everyone, and I think my sister and I were as disoriented and helpless then as at any other point. It was a whole new world we had to learn about, and through the whole time, to pretend to Mum that nothing was wrong, and that we were coping fine.

And Mum had nightmares; a lot of nightmares. She was terrified and didn't really know what was happening, particularly at night time. She'd totally forget things for the first time during the day, and she'd cry out several times a night, and one or both of us would go down to her bedroom to calm her, re-assure her, help her to the loo if needed, and hear her beg us to sleep on the bed with her, and not leave her alone. My sister sometimes did as Mum asked. I tried to go with tough love, staying as long as she needed whenever she called out, but saying I was only a shout away. I wanted her to be able to get through the night on her own. Desperately. I didn't want her to use us as a crutch and get so used to our presence that the night terrors might go on and on for her. At the same time I felt immensely guilty whenever I went back upstairs to leave her alone, like I was abandoning her. I'd lay awake when I went back upstairs, waiting for her to call again, ready to be there in an instant, but she never did.

I think the worst part during those weeks was seeing Mum so scared, so frail, so confused, and having to accept the conclusion that perhaps the Mum we knew had already gone and might never be coming back to us. It's a horrifying thing to admit to yourself, and only the fact that my sister was going through the same thing made it bearable. We weren't alone, and could share our fears. At the same time, a portion of our minds retained the worry that something inside of Mum still knew what was happening too, despite appearances, so we could never let our worries show in front of her; we just tried to act as if everything was perfectly normal. Even though those night terrors were nothing to do with us, it felt to me like they were, and the ever-present guilt wasn't just at returning to my bed after she'd had a bad turn, but more generally that we weren't (I wasn't) doing enough, or might be doing something wrong. There really isn't a manual. There is a strange 'twilight zone' feeling to every day, and somewhere at the back of your mind, you tell yourself that this is temporary, that it's only re-adjustment, but we really weren't sure if Mum would ever recover from those horrible, scary nights.

There were other adjustments we had to make too. As well as the necessary physical changes to the house (key safe, rail for getting in and out of the bath, higher loo seat so she wouldn't have to get up and down so much), we also had a 'falls alarm' installed. Absolutely bloody useless if you ask me. It would go off quite regularly, even when Mum wasn't moving at all and was sat in the chair next to me; suddenly, a disembodied voice would float through from the unit in the bedroom, asking if everything was okay. The one time it seemingly didn't work was when Mum had the fall that led to her death. That would be hilarious if it wasn't so tragic. They do have a button you can manually press for attention as well, but Mum being Mum, she'd never press that and bother anyone, even if she remembered it was there and what it was for. I'm not blaming the hardware exactly; we aren't talking about a sentient being, we're talking about a fairly low tech wireless motion sensor on the wrist, and I'm sure that for many it provides re-assurance, but given the fact that the calibration is next to impossible to get right, if it's something you're considering, I'd advise you not to rely on it too much. If a patient has the wherewithal to press the button when needed, or doesn't move their arms much, it might occasionally help, but if our experience is anything to go by, the number of false alarms would probably render the operator at the other end fairly blasé about regular calls from any particular house. A better idea was the bed sensor, tucked under the mattress, which could be programmed to raise the alarm if someone got up in the night and didn't return to bed, because they might have fallen or got stuck, though as Mum weighed about the same as an anorexic sparrow, it probably wouldn't have registered there either.

As I've said before, I'm a planner of worst-case scenarios by nature and, though it broke my heart to do it, I started investigating the possibility of a Care Home. My sister was dead against doing that so soon but I knew, from other people I'd talked to, that waiting lists can be long; months, years even; and I didn't want to risk reaching the point we'd have to place her somewhere that wasn't good enough, even temporarily. Despite earlier discussions with Mum (the abstract ones about how we should never give up our lives to look after her), both of us would have done that in a heartbeat, but my concern was that we wouldn't be enough. The way Mum was then, the nightmares, the fear, I didn't know if we'd be able to care for her long-term, which is a horrible thing to admit, but if she needed specialist round the clock care, neither of us was a health professional, and Mum's welfare had to come first. For me, even though it went no further than initial research and was an awful thing to do, feeling like a betrayal, researching potential Care Homes was one of the few practical steps I could take, so on balance I'm glad I looked. It may have helped to distract me and protect my sanity and, if nothing else, brought various questions to mind about care, medication and routines that would prove useful after the re-ablement team had gone.

Sometimes during these first weeks, Mum was almost like herself and we'd joke or watch TV like we used to before anything happened, but for most of the time she was quiet, scared, and nervous. The words "our Mum has gone" was a phrase we admitted to each other on more than one occasion, feeling totally lost ourselves. Fortunately, if slowly, Mum's panic and confusion started to lessen over the weeks, and while I kept a close eye on the Homes in the vicinity, I never got further than Googling and speaking to friends about their experiences with particular places.

What follows now is going to be another huge jump in the timeline, or how it felt, anyway. "Lessened over the weeks." Those four words to cover what was both an awful and a wonderful time, seeing sparks of Mum's return, sleeping through the night without calling for us, but at the same time seeing her limitations physically, and knowing they'd never completely go, that she'd never be able to do so many things she'd always taken for granted. Just watching her struggle with a Zimmer Frame was heart-breaking; this amazingly strong and active woman who, it seemed like only a few months ago, would tackle ladders and stairs with abandon. What mattered though, was that she was improving. With the best will and intentions in the world, we wouldn't have been able to cope at that point if she hadn't improved.

So gradually, and amazingly, Mum started to recover. It left its mark on her, and her confidence was completely shot but, day by day, the sense of 'our Mum' being in the building came back to us. Most of her, anyway. Some of the time you could almost imagine it was back after her first fall. She weaned herself off reliance on the Zimmer Frame sometimes, on her better days, and over time even went away for short trips with my sister once or twice, and we went shopping together (very carefully). This came alongside other improvements. It's amazing to think that all this, all these changes, the ups and downs, lowest of the lows and seeming recoveries, only happened over the course of a couple of years. Looking back, it feels like a decade.

At the same time Mum was starting to come back to us, we were presented with the fact that you only get six weeks from the re-ablement team; the hospital can't resource any more (not just for us, that's the policy), so we'd need to find private carers to take over those duties too.

Private care is very expensive, and if you're ever in the position of needing it, you'll likely to be shocked at just how expensive it seems. If you break it down to an hourly rate, and think about the level of responsibility, it really isn't an unreasonable amount, and the pay and conditions for those working there, even pre-pandemic, isn't good, but when you see the thousands per month you're paying out... well, have a stiff drink before you open the first invoice. I may sound harsh about some of the carers over the coming pages, but that's because there are two distinct aspects at play here. The state of the sector, government lack of oversight (lack of funding), and lack of training and support for the carers is one matter, and anyone who works in the sector has my unflinching support and admiration. But when you're caring for your ill parent, none of that is at the forefront of your mind. As expensive as it might be, all that mattered to us was ensuring the best possible care for Mum, and I'm afraid that if that meant being a fussy pain in the arse to the company providing the care, then that's what would happen. Staffing and training issues aren't my responsibility, and all I cared about was the company fulfilling its duty of care and looking after my mum. Some of the carers were incredible and we knew we could trust them implicitly with any situation. But some of the staff were either so long-serving that they were desensitised to individual patients' needs, and some others... well, let's just say they weren't well-suited to the vocation, and all they cared about was their hourly wage and clocking off as quickly as they could.

So, we thoroughly researched and found what seemed to be the best of the available local care companies, a set of questions drawn up between us to try and identify the most reliable and approachable, and then we invited a few round for Mum to meet, and to talk through what they did in more detail. There's a potential whole chapter in that round of meetings, and let's just say the level of support provided was variable, but this is about Mum's memory, not what the different companies we saw were like. Suffice to say, we chose a company we thought provided the best care and fit, and had them coming to help out four times each day; getting up and breakfast, lunch, teatime, and supper/ready for bed time.

My sister and me were still there too, as often as we could be, and we kept a close eye on the care Mum was receiving, very vocally pressing when it didn't live up to the standards we needed. Even before the pandemic, the private care sector could be problematic. There were no qualifications needed to be a carer, and there was inadequate pay and poor conditions for those working there. Some of the staff were really amazing and went above and beyond, and you could see the compassion. The others I mentioned, after seeing how they acted, we asked not to be assigned again, quite vociferously. You really need to keep an eye on what happens on the visits at first; that was one of the first lessons we learned.

The care plan we agreed with the company wasn't always followed in the early days, and some criteria were not always met. One, for example, was that we decided that for Mum's comfort (visits included help dressing and getting in and out of bed), there should be no male carers. Male carers can be just as good as female ones, but it was a decision we made together, as Mum was old school about some things, and with forgetfulness, the sight of a strange man who she didn't remember letting himself in to her bedroom as she woke up was something we wanted to avoid. I checked the visit logs the carers filled in on every visit each time I came back to see Mum, once a week at the very least, and monitored the timetables and rotas for who was due to arrive and when. I soon had to call up and complain when I discovered that a man made one of the visits. "He's very nice and very good" they said. "I don't give a fuck" was my admittedly blunt reply. If you agree something in a care contract, the company can't just change the agreement, and without letting us know, either. "We were short staffed." Again, not my problem. We pay a large amount of money for the agreed care. If you can't staff your rota, take on more staff from your profits and don't agree to things you can't deliver. Even with the best companies, you suspect the priorities that come down from 'on high' don't put compliance with agreed care plans at the forefront of the business model.

As I mentioned earlier, the title for this book came from the phone call refrain we made several times every day to Mum, to check who had turned up, if it was when they were supposed to come, and what they'd actually done when they were there. The issue with asking Mum about the visits of course, even when I later cross-checked against the logs for actual visit details, was that sometimes Mum would forget someone had been, even if they'd only left ten minutes before; other times she'd breezily say they'd already been when it turned out that no-one had arrived yet.

I think, if you end up in a similar situation, you should make a definite effort to read the carer logs for each and every visit. It's quite revealing in terms of who does what when they attend, what they actually record, and, by matching what they wrote against the times I'd phoned Mum, it was also useful for pointing out when carers had been or gone well outside the window of reasonable timekeeping, or the times they'd claimed they made the visit would have been while I was on the phone, and no-one was present. Turning up for the bedtime call at 7pm when it should be 10pm isn't acceptable, and was no use to Mum; nor is having the teatime call made at 3.30pm. There's also the issue, as I mentioned earlier, of Mum's tendency to 'not want to be a bother.' "No need to come back later," she'd try and tell the carers in the early days. Or she'd suggest she didn't need anything after all, and that they could go after five minutes, when they were supposed to be there for thirty. That was something that we had to watch out for, and we had to insist that any changes to visit lengths or cancellations were approved by me or my sister first. The fantastic carers would ignore Mum's mild objections anyway, but some of the less fastidious ones... well, they were simply happy to have an easy day and would take her at her word without question and leave or not return as they were supposed to, because she'd said it was okay. And I'm certain they knew damn well they weren't allowed to do that under the company rules either.

I should point out that, for much of the time, Mum was quite capable of fending for herself, feeding and dressing herself, and the point of the four times a day was to provide company and conversation for her, and to ensure (cajole) that she remembered to eat and do the things she should, to look after herself. They were a prompt as well as a practical help. Eventually she settled into the routine.

I should volunteer at this point, as an admission and in the spirit of openness, that I really fancied one of the carers too, and it was very hard not to flirt too much (as I think it might have been reciprocated). I don't mention this because it might be a more general hazard for everyone but, whatever memory or focus problems Mum had, I'm almost certain she was very aware of this attraction, and of course remembered that bloody fact, even if she'd forget everything else. Mums always know, and she'd make the occasional knowing reference to this one carer, with a twinkle in her eye. That was good to see, as it meant my mum was present and correct, observant and remembering things. Even if it was uncomfortable being teased when I was trying to ignore it and keep our relationship with the carers purely business.

I should mention, in case it's useful for anyone reading who might find themselves in a comparable situation, that there were quite a few other unexpected issues we hadn't even thought about, which also came up with the duties of the care company. It's easy to forget that most of their employees have no specific medical background, so there are limits, for instance, on what they're able to do with medication. One of Mum's meds, for example, was half a particular tablet daily. We hadn't thought it would be a problem but, for whatever reason, this pill wasn't able to be issued in a smaller dose, so had to be manually cut in half. The chemist had a huge waiting list for being able to deliver them pre-cut, and the carers themselves aren't allowed to undertake that task. It meant that, as prescriptions never end up with more than a day or so overlap, one of us had to schedule a visit over in a specific window (often midweek when we were both at work) for the sole and express purpose of taking a kitchen knife and halving pills. It doesn't sound like a big deal, and in the grander scheme of things, it isn't, but what can be the most tiring aspect of all this is keeping track of these small but essential tasks which shouldn't really have needed us, also untrained as pharmacists, to complete.

Another thing we put in the agreed "care plan," was that one of the purposes of the several visits was for company and chatting opportunities for Mum; we'd leave books, photos, memorabilia related to Mum's history, to be able to prompt this sort of conversation. But how do you tell if this side actually happens? With some of the ladies who came, this obviously worked a treat, and aside from Mum's enthusiasm for those carers, on the occasions one of us was there during the visits, it was easy to eavesdrop and find out what sort of interactions took place. Some barely said a word beyond what was necessary for meds/food, and in their minds the visits were purely practical in nature. Some, I know for a bitter fact after asking about activities, hadn't even read the care plan they were supposed to follow at all. This is one of the big down-sides of a commercial company. The re-ablement team comprised a small pool of carers who came regularly; once you move to an external company, you get whoever is available on the roster, who may even be travelling from a different area for a single visit. I don't blame the individuals for this, but as a business concern, the franchise clearly want to maximise efficiency and profits, so they build the rotas on that basis. The most work out of the minimum required employees. Some of Mum's regulars were fantastic and amazing, and clearly loved what they did, particularly interacting with the patients, but for others, it was a stop-gap job. We also had agreements in the care plan that they might, for example, encourage Mum to take a little trip outside to show off her back garden, to keep her mobile and stop 'outside' from becoming a no-go zone, or we'd leave jigsaws for them to do together. We quickly realised that the 'care plan' itself was only really useful for liaising with the company office, and left notes up in the kitchen suggesting things to do. This was very uncomfortable, and we needed to somehow balance Mum's self-confidence and natural pride in her independence, with the practical measures that might ensure she was getting better help. Mum didn't like the signs much, which would of course be visible if her friends came round too, but on balance it seemed the best, if not ideal, approach.

It might be unworthy of me, but there is always a fear at the back of your mind as well. You hear such horror stories in the press, from theft to mistreatment, and when carers you've never encountered before visit, that fear is greater. You've placed the one you love in their care but have no idea what they're actually like. You have to rely on the company's vetting procedures and training, and in the sector they seem so desperate for staff that you suspect it isn't always quality that wins out. The job adverts you see tell the story, "no experience necessary" being one of the headline non-requirements, which will naturally attract some who aren't cut out for the profession, but can't get other work.

Another of the elements we hadn't thought about enough was that you also have to consider and plan food quite carefully. Even in a 45 minute call, if we needed Mum to have hot food, we had to think practically. There isn't time to properly cook from scratch (and eat, wash up, etc.), so things that can be heated up were the preference, and we'd cook and leave home-made meals. Mum never liked microwave food, and the temperatures of ping-heated food are easy to burn mouths with, so we tried to avoid ready meals where we could, but the cooker itself took so long to heat up that the microwave meals were often the most effective solution, and we had to hope that whoever came had the gumption to actually check how hot something was.

Another aspect of care and comfort around food and drink that you can't account for in advance is personal preference. We (and the regulars) knew how milky Mum liked her tea, that she liked the cheese for her crackers cut quite thin (almost slivers) but a number of the carers wouldn't ask first and Mum, with her reticent nature, would be too polite to mention it, and would accept whatever was given with a smile, even though she might struggle with, or not enjoy what she was given. It was down to me or my sister to point out to a carer when we saw that Mum liked the cheese in slivers, for example, and we'd have to hope they'd remember and do things differently the next time they visited. We also had to hope that they would take the request in the manner it was intended, and not take offence, as who knows what that might result in. It was a constant fear and balance on how to talk to the carers. Always polite, but sometimes you need to insist on certain behaviours, and you don't want to risk your own tone offending the carer, with the risk that Mum might be on the receiving end. It never happened, as far as I know, and we took extra care, but it was another thing to fret over.

Dates of food are also something I'm very particular about personally, and in the early days, one of my regular obsessions was to check dates on bread and food in the fridge on my weekly visits. While it was part of the carers' defined tasks to check food dates, when you have four different people visiting in a day, some would just assume it would be the next person that would deal with the issue, and I'd find out of date food ready to be served up. When we cooked or prepared, we started using Tupperware and stick-on labels with opened and use by dates. Fortunately, we had a very good carer who came the most frequently in the morning, and who started to leave notes in the care log for the subsequent helpers, "If ham isn't used today, please put in compost bin," "please wrap cheese in clingfilm after use", etc. She was a godsend for peace of mind.

The Experience – The Funeral

I think I might do this last section in reverse and start with the funeral, if you don't mind. As you might guess, it's a difficult area to talk about but there's method in my madness (excuse the poor choice of phrase), as a number of choices we made for Mum's funeral (the music, the "do," the service) were particular references to Mum's later years. It's a hard balance, knowing how to plan a service and "the do" ("the wake" doesn't seem the right term for us, and I associate that more with religious funerals). We wanted to celebrate Mum's whole life, but the woman we were saying goodbye to right then needed to be central to the events. And... well, she wasn't quite the woman we grew up with.

Part of the planning was for the afterwards "do" playlist, back at our house after the funeral. My sister and I chose not just the music for the service, but also two CDs of music we could listen to back at the house, as background noise. The songs we chose wouldn't mean much to most of the people attending, who wouldn't even listen to most of that noise, to be honest, and we were quite aware of that. But the music we chose would mean something to us, would be about our relationship and history with our mum, and the planning of this would be a relatively light and "fun" (in the loosest sense) task for us to do together. The songs we chose couldn't be too downbeat, and we picked examples of music Mum loved, or that we shared a specific bond or memory over, and we talked about these together as we came up with the list of potential tunes.

The playlist was a real mixture. Some choices were songs that Mum had always loved herself; Joseph Locke, *Hear My Song*, and Pat Boone, *Love Letters in the Sand*, Michael Ball of course (she'd been in the fan club and had every recording he made, we went to concerts and everything in earlier days), and a lot of musicals (selections from *Phantom, Hair, Oklahoma, Godspell, The Lion King*) as Mum loved them, and we'd both been to live musicals with her too. We also had a selection from people and bands she used to go and see play live occasionally, Ken Dodd, The Houghton Weavers, Jacqui and Bridie. It was odd in retrospect, for a woman who always told us she was happy sitting in silence and didn't know why we always needed background noise, and who had relatively few records or acknowledged favourites, that we realised there was a lot of musical history. From the records she'd had when she was younger, we added Clinton Ford - *He Played the Ukulele As the Ship Went Down*, Harry Secombe - *We'll Keep a Welcome*, and the Glenn Miller Orchestra. One of Mum's favourite radio shows, *The Organist Entertains*, was represented by Reginald Dixon being 'beside the seaside,' and even the Beatles got a surprising shoutout, and an even more surprising choice, *Octopus's Garden*. I had absolutely no idea, but she'd once told my sister, related to hearing it, that this was her and Dad's 'song,' which is bizarre, but somehow also fits. I think there were snippets of wonderful history that came to light over these discussions, which we might never otherwise have shared, so there are positives too. I learned more about my mum in planning the music for her send off.

Other playlist choices were based on personal connections my sister and I had with Mum, listening to songs together. I won't detail all the reasons but, for my sister, this included Michael Ball doing *The Rose*, Tom Jones - *Green Grass of Home*, The Searchers' - *Needles and Pins*, and for me, Mel C's version of *I Don't Know How to Love Him*, Perry Como - *Magic Moments* and B.J Thomas - *Raindrops Keep Falling on My Head*. Two very special choices, which we'll come back to the reasons for, were Keith Michell - *Captain Beaky and His Band*, and Manfredd Mann's *My Name is Jack*; songs we'd quote relentlessly with Mum; a familiar and always (usually) remembered routine and fun exercise.

We listened to the CD we'd made ourselves in the days before the service, afterwards, and when we were packing up her house to sell later on. I still have the playlist on my PC and it makes a regular appearance. I have it on at the minute. It brings back happy memories now, not sad, and is a lovely way to remember all those different times with Mum.

The choice of music for the actual service was more difficult. You needed music appropriate for a funeral service and for the guests, things that Mum wanted or would have liked/ appreciated; but, most of all, they had to be 'right.' I doubt many people there understood our choices, but there were reasons for all of them. I think we thought that the funeral was the final thing my mum, my sister and I would share together, so the meanings between us were all that mattered. It's perfectly justifiable to be selfish with this music, I think, and I don't regret a single choice.

The three of us shared moments afterwards, too, the living two of us and Mum's ashes, anyway, 'watching' the

Queen's speech together, when she was scattered, when we've visited since. But at the time the funeral had seemed like the full stop, and we would plan for it to be the last special occasion we all shared.

John Williams' *Cavatina* was the music we chose to come into the crematorium to. Aside from it being a beautiful piece of music in its own right, and very seventies (a wonderful period of memories for us with Mum then, as we were both kids), there was another reason. In her last year we'd often sit in the lounge together in an afternoon or evening, and Mum would nod off to whatever music we put on, and on the odd occasion would pick a CD herself. The collected John Williams album was one of these and was pretty much guaranteed to send her off to sleep to pleasant music, so it seemed fitting.

The two funeral pieces Mum chose for herself, when we'd all made our Wills a few years earlier, were Psalm 23, and *Abide With Me*, both fairly traditional. My sister and I chose versions which had even closer links to each of us, and to our mum. The version of *The Lord is My Shepherd* was the Howard Goodall one, also the theme tune for *The Vicar of Dibley*. We'd both watched that with Mum, either originally when it first aired, or latterly on DVD, and in the final months I'd often watch an episode again with her. She didn't really remember what had happened in the episodes, though we'd watched them all several times by then, but they were short, pithy, had her cackling at the "Yes Yes Yes... No" catchphrase, and I'd make her laugh by always misquoting the title lyrics in the wrong order, loudly and out of tune. In her honour, I did that during the funeral service itself too, though I mimed it silently so as not to upset the congregation. I know she'd have appreciated that. The version of *Abide With Me* was the BBC National Orchestra of Wales one, to the traditional tune *Eventide* by William Monk, used in the modern version of *Doctor Who*. We watched that with Mum, and my sister had close connections to the show and the home of the National Orchestra, something Mum was immensely proud of. Our chosen final 'show closer,' which no doubt totally bemused everyone else present, was Stevie Wonder's *Isn't She Lovely*. We weren't sure what we should pick at first, but as we went through various options and ideas, listening to a variety of tracks, both my sister and I had started to cry when this came on, so it was a no-brainer. Every time I left Mum's to come back to my flat, we had an almost ritualistic routine of quotes we'd go through, as routine is always good for familiarity for people with memory problems, and after the quotes we'd recite (which I'll come to), she'd get to her feet, we'd hug and sway, and I'd sing *Isn't She Lovely* to her, ending "isn't she lovely, isn't she wonderful, isn't she lovely, my lovely, lovely Mum." It was the perfect way to say goodbye at the end of the service.

Another very special choice for the service was my sister reciting Keats' *Meg Merrilies*. If you're not familiar, it's the poem that starts "Old Meg, she was a gipsy, And liv'd upon the moors: Her bed it was the brown heath turf, And her house was out of doors." Mum used to recite this to my sister when she was a child, and had learned it with her own mum, and we'd included it in the 'This is Your Life' book we made for Mum's 70th birthday (more on that later). The poem holds very special memories, but also, lest I forget the

period of Mum's life we're talking about her
one.

In the year before Mum's death, my sister
poem off by heart, to recite back to her, echoing those
times when they'd shared the words. Sadly, Mum didn't
really register the meaning or effort when the time came for
it to be performed for her. It's one of those horrible
occasions where you try and do something special, and it
doesn't quite work out as you'd hoped. She'd smiled and
said she liked it of course, but the reaction was, maybe also
typical of Mum who didn't like showing too much emotion,
very much that of a woman who wasn't quite sure why it
was being recited, and didn't realise the significance, effort
and thought that had gone into it. Things like that are so
hard, and you can't blame or push someone to react when
the reason they don't is their illness. It was par for the
course. The book I mentioned, the 'This is Your Life', was
the result of six months' work between my sister and I,
contacting and tracking old friends and family and
photographs; writing and including reminiscences; having it
printed and bound as a proper hardback called "Primrose,"
the central Christmas gift that year. The reaction we got was
more along the lines of "Oh, that's nice, dear", and onto the
next present. Maybe Mum was a bit overwhelmed, but
underrated reactions were a hallmark of our mother, even
before she got ill. There's another whole book of anecdotes
that could be written about her underwhelmed reactions to
gifts and surprises.

At the funeral "do" after, we also had a custom jigsaw of
Mum for guests to put a piece or two in. Mum loved jigsaws,
though in the last year or two it was less and larger pieces,

with fairly weak eyesight and motivation, she was less ivested and, to the frustration of whoever was watching, would try clearly wrong pieces repeatedly, stubbornly not looking at the picture or recognising the wrong colours. We enjoyed the jigsaws too and it was difficult to try and make sure we didn't correct her or put too many pieces in ourselves, so that Mum felt equally a part of completing the puzzles. She loved them in general, though, and depending on the picture we chose (or got her to choose), would often have "old" scenes or brands that might provoke memories of her younger days.

During my 'bit' of the service, I took off my suit jacket and donned the Starsky and Hutch cardigan Mum had knitted for me, knowing she'd be slightly aghast, but secretly and wickedly proud that we'd given her a proper and serious funeral for the guests, but also that we did it 'our way.'

The Experiences - Vignettes

This chapter is more a series of vignettes and memories than a narrative, presented to you as events come back to me while I'm writing other sections, but I think they might be the most valuable part of this story too. And they may chime the most with anyone who has experienced a family member or friend on a similar mental descent. With any luck they will provide both hope and insight, and the occasional giggle, and, as well as giving examples of the bad times, will prove that there can still be wonderful experiences to come too. They are also a reminder that while, probably from the time of her first leg injury, our mum's physical and mental health deteriorated, the essence of the old lady remained, and even after the initial period when we thought we'd lost "her" totally, she came back to us, and right up to the day before she died, our funny, wicked, irreverent Mum was still there, peeking out occasionally.

Let's start with an equal parts terrifying and hilarious experience. Mum didn't like doctors, or rather was never relaxed or comfortable around them, and would use humour as a defence mechanism. We'd all be daft in awkward situations, as it defused seriousness, and helped us bond and feel a sense of togetherness, but in the latter years Mum's sense of the appropriateness of comments went out of the window. And she had a propensity to "joke" with doctors about how I'd lock her in a cupboard if she misbehaved, or put her in the bin (don't ask), or beat her up. I know, it doesn't sound at all funny out of context, but with people who knew us and knew that nothing could be further from the truth, it was a distracting 'joke type thing' for her to say. Similar to our "do as you're told or we'll put you in a home" comeback, the phrases sound horrible written down, but try to imagine them being said and received as a family joke; "Go and fetch me some cake or I'll lock you in the cupboard," "Right, that's it, I'm putting you in the bin" (lifting her up off the floor). Not particularly funny to anyone else but, as with any family in-joke, often hilarious to us.

Now that's fine to say amongst ourselves at home, but when we started with the re-ablement team, and with carers and other medical professionals, this type of joke started to take on a dangerous edge. It was still fine to joke around with the carers who came regularly and knew our dynamic and silliness, of course, but as I tried to gently point out to Mum, if a health professional hasn't met us before and hears a joke which is essentially about domestic abuse, they might be obliged to take it seriously, in case it's a genuine cry for help. I tried to gently chide Mum, asking her not to make those kind of jokes in the company of strangers, but the problem was that I didn't want to sound too serious and upset her, or perversely flag up the joking as being *too* significant, so that the idea might come back to her at inopportune moments. But at the same time I needed to try and make her understand the potential consequences; to get her to understand why she couldn't make those jokes any more. It was just that they were inappropriate things to say in those settings. But Mum didn't really get what my concern was. Plus, of course, with memory being the issue, if she did realise and say she was joking, she'd have forgotten by the next time she was talking to a doctor. And on more than one occasion when we were in hospital or at a doctor's consultation, she would try to lighten the mood, "I have to do what he says or he'll punish me and put me in the bin!" I would be mortified each time, worrying that something might be read into the throwaway attempt at humour.

The horror is that when all you want to do is wrap someone in cotton wool, there's a real danger that, if someone decided they needed to take Mum's joke seriously, we could actually be taken away from her, which would destroy her and, to add to that, she wouldn't understand why. Even more importantly, it could potentially result in her being separated from us, so that we couldn't look after her. Stupid bloody jokey approach to nervousness. I should add, in the interests of transparency, that the bin thing started when I was about 17 and taller than her for the first time. I'd just taken the rubbish out and, before putting a new binbag in, I told her, deadpan, that there was something else I needed to do. And I physically picked her up and carried her over to the empty bin as she struggled, laughing as she realised what I was doing, and placed her inside, in the place of a binbag. She wasn't that tall, and the bin came up to her hips, too high for her to climb over, so she had to try and be angry with me, between her own giggles, and command me to pick her up and lift her out again. I just stood and crossed my arms and said, "nope," grinning as she tried to be angry and failed, in the end saying I'd better lift her out, or if I made her keep laughing, she'd wet herself. And I'd be the one to clean up the mess. That was how it started. You only needed one occasion to start a running joke in our family. If I said, "I wouldn't mind, but it wasn't her bike", "Ooh look, it's raining," or "Jamaica" then you'd no doubt wonder what the hell I was grinning at, but one occasion each of those phrases was uttered by a member of our family led to decades of repeated jokes, which just got funnier with time.

My next memory isn't a happy one for me, but is a good example of several unfortunate interactions with Mum where she became very distressed and upset, and I vividly remember each one, though she'd be happy and smiling and have forgotten all about it an hour later. It informs the events of the story I've included at the end of this book, and is sadly typical of those occasions I can't forget, when I could do nothing to ease Mum's confusion and stress, and I felt totally helpless.

Mum was a bizarre mix of technophobe and technically adept. While smartphones would have been a step too far and we bought simple mobile phone handsets for her, Mum took to the concept and operation of mobile phones and texting like a duck to water, or a Yorkshire woman to cricket. Even the bizarreness of predictive text didn't really seem to faze her, though things got more difficult towards the end. The issue I wanted to mention though, was during a period between carer visits one afternoon, when I got a text from Mum while I was at work, saying that she couldn't get the television to switch off. Having had a few similar occasions when this had happened before, I phoned back straight away, knowing she'd be getting frustrated and would be winding herself up. Even in the periods when she struggled with memory or concentration, Mum was often aware and "with it" enough to recognise when a seemingly simple task just wouldn't happen. She'd know it was something she should be able to fix herself, and would get increasingly frustrated that she couldn't sort it out by herself. She'd get gradually more upset with that inability to solve the problem and, in a vicious cycle, the more upset she got, and the more flustered, whatever task she was trying to undertake naturally got even more difficult.

I should mention at this point that we do genuinely seem to be cursed in our family with idiosyncratic remote controls, and I'd encountered remotes that refused to behave for myself on numerous occasions, so it wouldn't have been anything she'd done herself which had caused the problem, though I knew she'd be blaming herself and thinking it was somehow her fault. For some unknown reason (and we tried various remotes over the years), sometimes the damned things just wouldn't work. There were usually two ways to fix this; fiddle with the batteries or turn the set off at the plug and then turn it on again. The latter would have been too difficult to explain and the kneeling and dexterity wouldn't have been possible. So it would probably be a case of rolling the batteries around in the back of the remote.

I assumed, as she'd managed to text without any problems, that Mum wasn't too upset yet, and we could fix it if I answered quickly, and stop her going into a cycle of confusion and stress. She was very apologetic and trying to sound calm when she answered, but the frustration must have been there for some time, and her seeming 'calmness' was a front, as her distress quickly accelerated. As she explained that she couldn't change the volume or turn the TV off, Mum got increasingly flustered.

I tried to talk through the possible fixes gently and conversationally, first checking that she was trying the correct remote (we had a blu ray player one, too) and she tetchily told me that of course she had the right one. Trying to be as calm as possible for her, I asked her to describe it anyway (we'd had her using the wrong remote before) and it sounded like the right one, but as I talked through where to point the device, and which other buttons to try pressing, she got even more agitated, assuming, I think, that she was doing something wrong, despite me telling her what to press. Sometimes other buttons work, so I had her describe where the green and red buttons were on the remote in her hand, so I could visualise what she was looking at. Her eyesight wasn't always brilliant with colours so I suggested she hold it up and close to look at the red button, and try pressing that, after which her voice got quieter and the line went dead. I knew instantly that she must have held up the phone handset instead and pressed the red button to turn that off, meaning our conversation ended. I'm sorry if this story seems long-winded, but it's only by understanding the steps we went through that you'll get the picture of what Mum did, and why she grew increasingly upset.

Mum would have been trying her best to follow my instructions to the letter, and would now be starting to really panic that, in addition to the original TV problem, I'd also inexplicably hung up and gone away, and that this might be her fault, too. I tried calling back but it was engaged, as she must have tried to press the buttons again and somehow blocked incoming calls. So I phoned the landline. I knew she'd probably have to struggle to get up out of her chair to reach it, but there wasn't really another option.

Mum managed to answer, but was in full-on panic mode; apologising, muttering and I suspect crying a little, and wasn't really listening to a word I said, so I did what you sometimes have to do, though all the advice is never to do this. I had to shout.

"Mum... MUUM... MUM.... LISTEN....LISTEN TO ME... JUST LISTEN A MINUTE... MUM!"

I finally got her attention and switched to talking as softly as I could once she was listening again, re-assuring her that everything was fine, and told her I was sorry for shouting (thankfully, she said she didn't realise I had) and talked her down. I reminded her that, in the big scheme of things, the television being on didn't really matter, the carer would be there within the hour and could fix it if we couldn't, we could try again if she wanted but didn't have to. Mum was nothing if not stubborn and determined and, having calmed a bit just from being talked to, she managed, as I gave directions, to slide the battery compartment over, roll the batteries, put the cover back on, and press the off button. It worked perfectly. She apologised for being silly which I said she wasn't, it was the remote's fault, which got a laugh. We talked for a few minutes and I told her I'd call again in an hour, after work. When I did, she barely remembered what had happened at all. For her it had been an "in the moment" panic, getting flustered because she was winding herself up about not being able to do something that should be simple.

On later occasions when we talked about getting a new remote, Mum half-agreed that it would be good, but whether she was feigning memory of the incident, or genuinely remembered, I don't know. The problem for me is that I was left with multiple guilts. One, that she was on her own (even for short periods) and had no-one to re-assure her; sometimes she seemed so fully in control it was hard to reconcile with the times she really wasn't okay. Second, I'd shouted at my mum. Even if she didn't remember, and it had been the right call and had worked (without it she'd likely have accidentally hung up again, as had happened before). Third, what would happen if she didn't manage to text or reach anyone? She was a practical woman and would probably have gone for a lie down on the bed, upset, but woken and either not remembered or been calm enough to deal with it herself. Fourth, and the main one when caring for a family member; I'm not doing enough for her and had let her down, it was my fault. Though I hated doing it, I found myself imagining her side of that afternoon, and that was part of the genesis for the short story you'll read at the end of this book. I can recall every moment of that phone call now, and I suspect I will always be able to, whether I want to or not.

The routine before leaving Mum's home at the end of a visit or staying over is the next memory that comes strongly to mind. I mentioned earlier that we had a ritual before I left the house every time, and this was built on a number of songs and rhymes we'd repeat, some which she'd repeat, and some from things she just inexplicably remembered very clearly. The first two of these were songs.

Captain Beaky was a spoken word children's' song that had been hit in 1980, and which I'd loved as a kid. The beginning goes... "The bravest animals in the land were

110

Captain Beaky and His Band, there's Timid Toad, Reckless Rat, Artful Owl and Batty Bat". I don't know why, but Mum (mostly) remembered all the words to that song, right up to her last days. The second tune, which was a bizarre choice, was Manfred Mann, *My Name Is Jack*. We were listening to *Pick of the Pops* on Radio 2 one Saturday afternoon in the last year of her life when it came on and, word perfect, Mum sang along to the whole thing. I was flabbergasted. Mum loved her music - folk, musicals, easy listening, etc., but pop music, particularly 60s pop music? *Really* not her thing. But she seemed to know the entire bloody thing, never having once sung it in my hearing in the previous five decades. One of the cruellest peculiarities of dementia is that patients frequently, and increasingly, have very poor short term memory, but the longest term memories often come back. Alongside this, there are some things they can no longer retain, and for no discernible reason; others they have an almost crystal clarity on. This turned out to be really useful. Feeling in control is re-assuring for anyone, but when you're vulnerable it's even more important, so at the times I was leaving Mum's house, I'd use things I knew she'd remember, little tasks I knew she'd achieve, to give her confidence, so it would both distract from me going and put her in a positive frame of mind about her own recall and capabilities. These were the first two songs we recited together in the routine when it first started. Over the weeks and months, the leaving ritual grew and grew though, and towards the end there were multiple elements and references; all things I knew she enjoyed and might be able to join in with.

You remember how I said a part of the memory assessment team test was telling someone a name and address, and later seeing how much of the detail they could recall? As I said, over the following days and weeks, I kept prompting Mum to try and recall that address, and through repetition, and familiarity, it became a fun 'game' to keep doing, with Mum quite happy to take part, as the more she recited the address, the more the details got drilled into her and the more it re-assured her she was capable of retaining information. And we realised this was a really useful tool for giving her confidence. That was what inspired this leaving ritual, which ended up so long that I'd need to start before I made a phone call for a taxi, as the car would undoubtedly have turned up halfway through our routine. This is how it ended up:

When it was time to go, I'd begin with a childhood rhyme of hers that Mum had recalled one day and then would repeat to anyone who'd listen, quite frequently.

There is a rude version as well, but essentially the one we told went, "Not last night but the night before, three tomcats came knocking at my door. One had a fiddle, one had a drum, one had a pancake stuck to his thumb (sometimes bum or tum)".

Don't ask me why, but Mum loved to repeat this bloody rhyme. A lot! I think it became a particular touchstone for her, something she knew she always remembered and shared with us. No idea why it came back to her, but by the end it was wedged so firmly in her memory that she'd trot it out at any given opportunity, several times a day. I think her carers knew it by heart after a few weeks.

Anyway, I'd start my leaving ritual with a question to ask her about what might have happened to her "last night," to set her up for the reply... "Well... not last night, but the night before…" And we'd go through questions and answers for the whole rhyme. "What happened then, Mum?" "Well, you'd never guess it but three Tomcats came knocking at the door!" "Did they really, were they carrying anything with them?" "Well, funny you should ask, but actually one had a fiddle!" "Really? Just the first one?" "Yes, but the second one had a drum!" etc. etc. It was more than just telling the rhyme; it was a shared comedy routine, and it was familiar and calming to her, and fun for us to play about with the back and forth, tweaking the questions and order each time.

Then, when we'd finished the Tomcats rhyme it would be onto 'Captain Beaky,' "Now Mum, before I go, remind me again, who ARE the bravest animals in the land?" She'd pretend to think, and then recite the lines from the chorus of the song, "Well, the bravest animals in the land were Captain Beaky and his band." "Really, and who was in this band?" Sometimes there would be slight inaccuracies, her giving "Ratty" for "Reckless" Rat, or "Ollie Owl" for "Artful Owl", but with a bit of prompting she'd always get there in the end and complete the lyrics, and I think there was a real pride for her that she'd remember each time.

Next, I'd ask, "Now, how, Mummy, HOW… do you THINK…the unTHinkable..?"

The origins of this very corny joke were in another family story, about a relation with a lisp who didn't seem to realise that they had a lisp at all. Sometimes she'd get the answer to that one, sometimes not, but she'd always laugh at the punchline, "WiTH an EYETHberg" (read the joke out loud to yourself, and imagine the lines spoken with a lisp, and you'll get the awfully bad joke).

Then it would be time for a Bullseye (TV show) catchphrase reference, and I'd do an impression of the compere Jim Bowen - "Very good, you've done very well so far, and your money's safe... but now, to win the speedboat... answer this... what's your name?"

This was when we'd do a back and forth version of the chorus from the Manfred Mann song, and she'd answer "Jack," invariably with a grin, enjoying the routine and ritual now, and confident she knew what was coming next. I'd interview her about the lyrics.

"And where do you live, Jack?"

"In the back!"

"Of what?"

"Of the Greta Garbo Home for wayward Boys and Girls!"

For whatever reasons, these song lyrics were so deeply ingrained that Mum never missed a beat in answering, or ever made a mistake.

"And are you a wayward boy or girl, Jack?"

"Yes."

I love things which seem 'meant to be,' and shortly after Mum's funeral, as I was taking some items to Oxfam to drop off, I found myself browsing and, at the front of the twenty or so 7" singles they had at the shop, there at the front was the very Manfred Mann single. I bought it and treasure it.

Finally in our goodbye ritual, it was time for a hug. Mum would struggle to her feet (I always let her do that for herself without assistance, so she was being capable and independent at the very end of the visit), and we'd deliberately shuffle towards each other, arms out as we approached. No idea why we shuffled, maybe I did it to mirror her and make it part of the game.

And once my arms were round her, I'd kiss the top of Mum's head and sing the chorus of Stevie Wonder's *Isn't She Lovely* to her, with the changed lyrics about her being my "lovely, lovely Mum" at the end, and swaying so it was a little dance as I sang. That was why we picked it as the final song for the funeral, too.

It was a beautiful way to leave the house each time, and made me feel better too. The day before Mum died, just before she went for her operation, not caring who was listening, my sister and I did the 'three tomcats' verse in the hospital out loud and she joined in, happy to be silly with us in public. And without us having to undertake an overly emotional 'this might be the final goodbye,' it let us do part of the leaving ritual with a smile. Just in case she didn't come back.

One peculiar little practice I started a number of years back, and I'm not even sure exactly what prompted it, a suggestion in a book maybe, was signing off all loved-ones' telephone conversations with the phrase "see you soon, love you lots." It may have seemed strange to them at first but fortunately, it caught on with the family and became automatic for the end of every phone call we made. The inspiration I don't recall, but the reason I do. Even before Mum got ill, it occurred to me, possibly in relation to the dying words my dad never got to say to me, that you never know when you'll lose someone. It was a half-jokey colloquial phrase I came up with, but the driver was simple. If anything ever happened to Mum, the last words we would have said to each other were, "see you soon, love you lots." Even if it had been a grumpy conversation for some reason, it had ended with that. We didn't need it, as it turned out, but it meant we said "I love you" hundreds of times a year, which is no bad thing in itself. I don't know if she ever realised why. Maybe, she wasn't daft. But she certainly wouldn't have known or remembered why we said it in the end. She'd just know that she'd hear she was loved every day from me and from my sister, and would always say it back. I'm so pleased that happened.

Even at the worst of times, there was both humour and pride in my mum. What follows is an example of both, I think. There are invariably a number of co-incidental medical issues that come with age, and one in particular comes to mind, from a few months before the end. Piles, and the use of bum cream! I'm sure Mum wouldn't mind me mentioning it, as it's the kind of story she'd have delighted in knowing and I can almost hear her cackling merrily over the story now.

Mum would genuinely forget some tasks and details but sometimes, I'm certain, she also used to use the dementia and memory issues as an excuse to avoid anything she didn't fancy doing. She was canny like that. It reminds me of how my grandfather (her dad) acted. Well before he was ill with Parkinson's, he would suffer from 'selective' illness' himself. I can remember him well, sat in his lounge and, to the complete belief of his wife and daughter, starting to suffer from loss of hearing; not answering to things they'd call through from the kitchen, oblivious to requests to do chores or help out. It reached the stage that they just accepted his 'deafness' and stopped asking him for help. At the same time, his hearing was miraculously perfect whenever he and

I chatted, or if it was me who was calling to him from another room, so long as there weren't female voices that might overhear. Slight digression there, but it's possible that this 'selective' illness might run in the genes.

So, in those months, when I'd be there in an evening, one of the prompts I'd frequently make when Mum returned from the bathroom was the reminder "did you remember to use your bum cream?" Mum would pause her walker a little way into the room (knowing what was coming next) and confirm that of course she had. So I'd ask again, "Did you *really* just use your bum cream?" to be met with an exasperated "Yes!"

I'd barely need to start "Mum, did you *really*... use" before she'd have turned the walker around to head back to the bathroom, grumbling at being caught out and then re-appearing a few minutes later. I'm willing to put good money on the fact on some of these occasions, she simply went to the bathroom and stood there, counting to fifty, thinking "I'll cap the little bugger" and refusing, on principle, to use or even look at the medication that was meant to help her, stubbornness beating all. When she returned there was no point in asking again, as I knew she'd fib but, as she'd seemingly done as asked, couldn't really be challenged on it. I was proud of her for that. It showed "she" was still there, in all her glory, wily enough to outfox anyone if she could, rebellious just for the sake of being rebellious. On the odd occasion it would be a game of chicken, and I'd let her hear me moving in the hall when she was in the bathroom, and she'd have to decide if she could risk standing and faking the application of the cream, as the door would always be slightly ajar in case of falls. Or I'd put the tube of cream just

117

inside its box knowing she never bothered to place it back in there, so I could 'accidentally' challenge her when I used the bathroom after her that it somehow hadn't left the box, despite her having just squeezed it. It doesn't sound like a fun game, but it actually was sometimes, for her too I think, with the occasional little pinched face expression or sticking her tongue out at me when it was obvious I'd caught her out in a fib, or the almost-imperceptible bland smile that showed she thought she'd got one over on me.

Other experiences weren't so much fun, and one particular memory really haunts me to this day and fills me with guilt, although I know I did nothing wrong. Often, Mum wouldn't want to go to bed at all, and would be really happy if my sister or me were staying over for the night and watched TV or listened to the radio with her, giving her an excuse to stay in her chair doing crosswords till midnight or after. For an unknown reason, on this particular evening when I was staying over, she clearly didn't want to go to sleep at all. Maybe she'd had nightmares when she napped during the day, maybe she was worried about settling, we'll never know. But I was really tired myself and I headed up to my bedroom about eleven pm. Mum was in her PJs with all the night-time tasks completed; I'd closed the windows and curtains, checked the door was locked, her hot water bottle was warming her bed and there was a glass of water by her bedside table, and I knew Mum was quite capable of heading to the loo and getting under the duvet herself. We always thought that her keeping a sense of independence was important to her, and to us too, so I kissed her goodnight and headed upstairs, gently suggesting she didn't stay up 'too late', not wanting her to spend the night in the chair having nodded off. I got up for a pee sometime after half-twelve and noticed that the light was still on downstairs, so went to check all was okay, and she was still sat in her chair, puzzle book on her lap. I asked if everything was okay, and she was obviously aware why I'd come down. I don't know if she'd had a little snooze and a bad dream again, but the figure in the chair wasn't a woman in her eighties, it was an insecure child. She looked up at me, seeming to be a bit guilty, and in a tiny voice, asked me, "Do I have to go to bed now?"

It was haunting, and crushing, and has woken me up on many nights since, seeing her like that, being treated, quite openly, like I was the parent; her voice a mixture of acceptance that she'd do whatever I told her to, but almost a pleading that I might say "no". I gave her a massive hug and, trying not to appear too emotional, told her that of course she didn't, I just wanted to make sure she was okay, but she really shouldn't stay up *too* late. I went back upstairs but didn't sleep, and heard her make her way to her bed about twenty minutes after that. But I still didn't sleep. I don't think she remembered at all in the morning but I did, and that memory has stayed with me. She was like a scared little girl, and I was so worried I'd cry in front of her and upset her, or let her down by not being strong, that I'd made my excuses and left, telling myself that I was helping her by letting her make the final decision herself. And all I wanted to do was hug her and stay there holding her, making her feel safe. That decision is still with me now. I wish it wasn't.

As a sidebar here, I also managed to load myself with an additional guilt, unrelated to our own situation, but proving that you can always learn and act better to people who have mental health difficulties. This revelation and guilt didn't occur to me until I was in my late forties, but it was only when I experienced Mum's deterioration and became carer for that I realised how some people must look through the lens of children, and how badly I'd behaved when I was one. In the early eighties I briefly had a job at the shops at the top of Mum's road, as a paperboy. And there was always one visitor to the shop who would invariably amuse me and my workmates.

I don't know who first termed her 'Mad Annie,' but there was an elderly lady who lived nearby who would frequently call in to the paper shop about 7am in the morning, before we opened, and as we sorted the papers, to ask the proprietor to wind her watch up for her. She'd turn up in her slippers and nightdress, seeming dazed, and would answer to the cruelty of the boys politely greeting her with, "Morning, mad Annie!" with a kindly smile and nod, oblivious of the insult, before shuffling off home. The memory of her came back to me as Mum came through from the bedroom one morning, half-asleep and a bit dopey. It hit me then, that while she never reached that level of bewilderment, there was quite possibly a family of 'Annie' who had no idea she took morning walks to the shops in her nightwear, clearly in no fit state to cross the roads safely, or deal with anyone she met. And we'd found it hilarious and were rude to her.

As I watched Mum shuffling through to the lounge one morning, I couldn't help imagining being Annie's son and walking into the paper shop to find her one morning, frantic that she was missing from her house. He would have seen how she was treated, and realised this was a regular routine for his mother. I don't mean to be patronising, as children don't know any better, but I wish to God I'd been nicer to Annie now, and not joined in. I've thought about her numerous times since. And 'Annie' may not even have had a family who were local, who cared, or may have never had children. So I think she deserves a place in my book too, to say I'm sorry Annie, and it have come decades too late, but you've taught me a lesson about thinking more before I speak, and what might lie behind seemingly amusing or oddly-behaving people. So thank you, Annie, and I'll try and pass on your lesson here

There are other anecdotes which didn't become known until much later, after Mum had gone, and conversations with family and friends brought back other memories for all of us. One was from Mum's good friend and neighbour, who would call round daily, provide company and emotional support, and whatever else was needed. Wonderful woman. But a couple of years later, she recounted to me how, when Mum sometimes decided to go to bed early, she'd ask her friend to go into the bedroom first, and look behind the curtains for her. Whatever it was in Mum's mind will remain an eternal mystery, as she never explained the reason, but apparently it happened numerous times. Maybe it was a return to childhood fears like monsters under the bed, and we'll never know, but I've thought about it many times since I found out. My best guess is that perhaps one night there had been a wasp or bluebottle which had startled or scared Mum with an unexpected appearance. Or maybe curtains had been closed and as she lay in bed the sound unnerved her, and prompted nightmares? I wish I knew, but I hate knowing there must have been times, without us or her friend there, that my mum was scared or worried. I almost wish I didn't know.

In the last years I started leaving my mobile phone on all night, on my bedside table, always half-expecting the horror of a midnight or early morning phone call from Mum in a panic. Mum never called during those hours, but because I left the phone on (and I'm inept with mobile technology so couldn't apply any clever settings), I'd often be jerked awake with a buzz or ring of notification of texts from other people who were more night owls, and my instant reaction every time was always abject fear that the buzz or ring would be about my mum. A couple of years later, I eventually worked out how to set silent hours, with exceptions for my sister's number or my mum's, but I never used it while Mum was alive, and never even thought about researching how. I reasoned that, even if I managed that, a call might come from neighbour, carer, or the hospital, and I couldn't take that risk.

It was such a strange experience after Mum died, having the mobile on silent and knowing I wouldn't be disturbed by my phone during the night, and for months I'd find myself checking the handset when I work up in the middle of the night, just in case there was something I'd missed, the action then automatic and, half asleep, not even remembering she was gone and nothing that came through could matter anyway.

They say that as dementia develops, the short term memory melts away, but long term memories come back, and this was certainly the case with Mum. Music can also be an extremely useful tool for provoking memories and providing comfort, and in recent years there is an increasingly acknowledgement of the benefits of song in research and in the public eye, with the idea of projects such as group 'dementia choirs' growing in popularity, bringing sufferers together for communal singalongs. These projects are all well and good if the sufferer is of an outgoing nature, or if their condition is so advanced that it is only the music itself that brings them back to life. Mum wasn't that far gone and. as you can probably imagine by now, she wasn't the sort of lady to join a choir with strangers, and I don't think she had sung in company outside family since Sunday school. But that didn't mean that music couldn't have similar beneficial effects.

In the final year, we'd reminisced about some of the nursery rhymes Mum used to tell us, and she'd sung along (with me) to *Donald Where's Your Troosers* and half-remembered couplets from *The Lion and Albert* when we'd listened to them on a Radio 2 programme (the latter lyric, if you don't know it, was a Stanley Holloway monologue-poem that had been recited to us as children). I made a decision and bought us a five CD set called *100 Hits - Children's Favourites (100 timeless nursery rhymes and songs)*. I was a bit apprehensive to be honest, not knowing if Mum might be offended or realise what I was doing, and the fact that they were listed as "Children's Songs" made me painfully aware, once again, that the balance of responsibility had shifted, and it was our turn to be the ones making the decisions. The CD wasn't all nursery rhymes and children's songs; there were tracks from musicals and older hits on there too, songs by Danny Kaye, Max Bygraves, Alma Cogan, Rosemary Clooney and Pat Boone, singers Mum had known when she was younger. These were alongside singalong favourites like *Puffin Billy*, *The Runaway Train*, *Run Rabbit Run*, *There's a Hole in my Bucket* and *My Boomerang Won't Come Back*. It worked a treat, and the CD would often be on in the background or we'd join in and sing along together now and again. I don't want to mislead you, Mum fortunately wasn't at any sort of regressive state, and most of the time we could speak about pretty much anything, adult to adult, and she'd surprise me with her recall of geographical or literary answers to crossword questions. We could talk about old family tree and family history matters and often she'd be sharp as a pin, so it wasn't that Mum had completely lost her faculties. Repetition and familiarity are re-assuring and comforting though, comforting at the best of times for anyone, but I'll say again, if you put yourself in the shoes of someone with memory issues, they can be an anchor. Mum retained enough awareness to know that words and facts sometimes eluded her, and even if she forgot specifics of the dementia, she was quite aware that she couldn't remember seemingly simple details. So finding an activity where you have recall and can join in, words you can grip on to, and know you will be able to participate as an equal. Well, those sorts of activities are invaluable. That's why old, familiar, tunes and TV help so much. The actual recalling of lyrics or singing along is secondary to the comfort of familiarity and sharing they bring, without feeling in any way less capable than anyone else in the room. When we had visitors (or the carers) and the CD played, it would be background noise and mostly ignored, or Mum would raise her eyebrows comically at the music I'd bought, putting on a front of "what is he like, playing this?" and keeping up a façade that it was all about me. And then, an hour later, she'd be happily reciting the words to the *Banana Boat Song*, not caring how 'grown up' the music choice was, just enjoying the singalong. Having the CD was an enormous success.

It helps that our family sometimes has a very juvenile sense of humour, and always has had. Since being 'amusingly childish' is something I'd always done on occasion (at least I thought it was amusing), this became a real advantage during that last year. Me being childish, be it via music, rhymes, or mock exasperation at impossible cryptics Mum could easily complete, meant activities like listening to the CD didn't come across as being all for her benefit either, or at least I hope they didn't. As we'd always enjoyed being slightly childish, it didn't seem too much of a change when it was done with the purpose of providing her with comfort, repetition and familiarity. I'm no expert, but being silly sometimes, in addition to the joy it brings to anyone, can be a useful pre-curser to activities for dementia sufferers. If the introduction of rhymes, songs and games is gradual, it doesn't seem to the patient quite so much like condescension, as though they're being demeaned. There's less risk of pride being offended, and it can also be fun and a stress reliever to patient and carer alike.

And the CD? I still have it and play it occasionally. It makes me smile, and remember fun times with Mum, even during the last weeks of her life. I think I'll always listen to it occasionally, for as long as I live.

It's true that our little family may have taken this approach to being juvenile a bit further than most. We have a three-inch finger puppet called Badger (guess what sort of animal it is), which has accompanied Mum on many holidays over the years (and been the star of photographs). This goes back decades, and we have an extended family of soft toys, which are literally our family too; some at my sisters, some at my flat, some lived at Mum's, and they'd all come together with us for events like Christmas. The toys have outfits knitted by my sister and mum (including a *Starsky and Hutch* cardigan for Floppydog to match the one Mum knitted for me, tanktops and socks for others (they're quite spoiled), but BeanieBum was the toy that lived at Mum's and was hers. I was gifted Floppydog by a housemate when I was in my early twenties (I was moving out and she wanted me to adopt him as a reminder of the good times we'd shared), and he was so soft and cuddly that my mum and sister kept trying to nick him, so about 20 years ago I had to get them their own versions, Beanie and Squashie. But I'm getting off-topic. Each toy had (has) their own distinct personality, with Mum's (Beanie) being an innocent, actually quite camp (big friend of the Musicals and Strictly), needy and wanting hugs. I'm not sure who was projecting what in his persona. He'd frequently sit on the arm of Mum's chair, reading with her (or looking at the pictures anyway; he was a bit too thick to be able to read!). We have folders full of photos of her sat in the chair or in her bed with the stuffed toys.

Having the toys and pretending they were interacting was a juvenile but harmless family pastime, but again was quite helpful in the last years. Even when Mum was alone in the house, she had a familiar presence nearby, almost a security blanket, and when we phoned, we could ask what Beanie was up to, and have fun with the answers. Let me make it clear that this wasn't done in an infantilising way; Mum was quite aware it was a silly conversation about a stuffed toy. But having distractions which didn't require serious discussions, the necessity of remembering anything, and could just be pure 'fun' were incredibly helpful in relaxing her. There would be no expectations, just messing about with her (admittedly grown-up) children, which might have brought back happy memories of when we were young too. Mum loved kids, and as neither me or my sister have spawned, it gave her the opportunity play-act the granny she never became and always wanted to be. Parenthood isn't for me, but I'm sometimes sad I wasn't able to give her that gift, and that she had to make do with the furry grandchildren instead.

We did other things which might seem odd, but which were just for fun, too. When Mum was in her mid-seventies, I think, I suggested we have a family Christmas in the middle of Summer, as there was no reason we should have to wait twelve months to enjoy turkey, sprouts and Carols. Initially, she was quite suspicious and was convinced I'd discovered that one of us had a terminal illness ("What do you know?" was her first reaction), but once she realised it was just for fun, we did exactly that. Cards, presents, crackers and Christmas Carols in July. I like that memory as it reminds me of how much fun our family was; unconventional maybe, but what the hell. Why not?

Another positive memory which comes back to me now is about bins. No, don't get excited, it may not be as thrilling as you hope. And it's more of a tip for you, actually, if you have an elderly and infirm parent yourself. If you're not aware (and I hadn't been), most local Councils have voluntary options to help the housebound. It might sound insignificant to you, but taking the bins and recycling boxes down to the side of the road for collection is one of those small but regular tasks which can be difficult to undertake if you don't live nearby. It is something that we discovered carers won't do (health and safety), and we couldn't really ask neighbours to do it for Mum every week, so were delighted when we discovered that this was a service the Council offered on request. After some initial cockups with arrangements (nothing is ever straightforward, is it?), the binmen came and fetched all the bins weekly from the side of Mum's house, without them having to be wheeled and carried down the drive to the grass verge.

My sister and I made sure we weren't in sight at collection times if we were staying over, just in case they saw us and removed the pickup, thinking someone capable was actually there; with my sister at the far end of country and me in work twenty-five miles away, without a car, we couldn't put them out ourselves every Tuesday morning. It was bittersweet to discover this wonderful service that the Council offers, and at the same time to remember that the real beginnings of Mum's illnesses and major health scares began because she was putting the bins out for herself and slipped on the drive.

While I'm on matters we arranged, we also bought Mum a new motorized armchair, one of those that can tip you upright, or raise your legs and lay you back. She didn't use it as intended unless we encouraged her, but keeping her legs raised was important for her circulation, so we tried to persuade her to do that whenever we visited. Mum hated all change but her previous chair was worn out, the springs gone, and we were at the stage where anything we could do for her comfort was done. Also, I think, it gave us something practical to be able to do ourselves helped us to feel like we'd made a difference. It wasn't in service long before we lost Mum, but here's another hint for you as we found out something which we, and I suspect many other people, didn't know. After Mum died, we had no further use for this bulky, practically new bit of furniture, so we donated it to one of the bigger local charity shops. These chairs aren't cheap, they cost several hundred pounds, but we found out that charity shops will often have them donated from situations like ours, and then sell them for a fraction of the retail price you'd pay for a new one. If you've looking for a new chair for a relative, it's worth bearing in mind that your local charity shop will probably have a number of practically new ones at a tenth of the price. It sounds a little icky and morbid to mention, but care is an expensive business, and this could be a significant saving, which also results in a charity making some money, rather than a commercial company.

I mentioned earlier that when Mum was seventy, my sister and I made her a 'This is Your Life' book. We got it professionally printed and bound (lots of companies do this now) and it was filled with photos, reminiscences of friends and family, poems, history, so a great life story for us to enjoy too. As I said, Mum's reticent nature meant her reaction was distinctly of the underwhelmed variety, but she did show it to friends and family, proud of what her children had done for her, as much as of what was in it, I think. But as the dementia took told, a decade later, the book proved to be a fantastic tool for prompting Mum to talk about and remember her life, with the carers who came, and also with my sister and I in the last years, when new details resurfaced and we found out new things about Mum which we'd never known. As short-term memory faded, longer term memories came back, and we'd find ourselves regaled with stories we'd never heard before, of neighbours, friends and even earlier pre-Dad boyfriends.

When Mum died, we initially had the idea of doing an updated version of the book, covering the following 12 years; I even set up a website for ideas and we announced it in the funeral programme and at the service, inviting contributions. We didn't get any, and the idea was slowly abandoned. I suppose it seemed strange to people, the idea of talking about Mum when she'd been ill, sharing stories of her at the stage when many of the stories would provoke more sadness than cheer. And the hard truth is also that she wasn't there to enjoy the memories and, with neither my sister nor I having kids, who would it actually be for? No-one really. On one level, this book might be what I was aiming for when the idea first came up. The original 'This Is Your Life' book is our story of our Mum's life before and with us, and this fills the gap of those later years, in a way that some other people might find insightful.

I'm going to incorporate a couple of short pieces here which we included in the original 'This Is Your Life' book. They take the form of two quite inconsequential rhymes (and they aren't any more than that), which I made up at the time to amuse my mum. They're essentially doggerel, with family memories crowbarred into couplets, but as we'd outlined Mum's influence on us, and things we did, I had to put some poems in, really. Mum inspired my love of reading and writing, which set me on the path to becoming an author, even if the things I wrote weren't really aimed at her, and poetry for me was always more of a side-line than a true vocation.

The amusing truth is, the very first time Mum heard one of my poems on the radio, she wasn't very impressed at all. I heard her on the phone afterwards, saying "it's very nice, but wasn't really a poem. It didn't rhyme." So it seemed important that anything I wrote for her book should foremost be a set of rhyming lines, and literary merit wasn't relevant. I was fine with that; after all, the book was intended for her entertainment, not for any self-aggrandisement. So I gave her what she would have expected of my writing rather than what I'd think of as poetry. That follows later.

I should add here that Mum was by no means unappreciative of all forms of poetry. She had books of it by Auden, Betjeman, Milne, and liked Keats and lots of classics. But if I created a poem, it should rhyme. That was her rule. They were proper and famous authors, geniuses, so could get away with whatever they wanted, but I was her son, so anything I wrote should rhyme and then she could show it off as 'proper' poetry!

"Primrose," by way of explanation, was my grandfather's nickname for my mum when she was a child. If you're wondering why I included such odd terms in these verses, they're puns and allusions to the family.

Primrose

If I could pick a Primrose, I'd try to resist.
They're naturally perfect just as they are,
They're beautiful and they perk you up,
The best of the flowers by far.

If I could pick a Primrose, I wouldn't.
They're precious and special and true.
They love the ground they live in,
But never forgot where they grew.

But if I *had* to pick a Primrose,
And I don't say that I would,
I'd choose a steadfast, green stemmed bloom
With roots still crowned in Mudd.

I'd want a vibrant, thriving flower,
Mature and full of vim,
Just coming to its blooming peak,
Un-secateured and trim.

I'd want a pretty, petalled head,
That's just a little grey,
That's lived, and knows a thing or two,
With anecdotes to say.

I'd want Anne extraordinary Primrose
That brightens up my day,
But if instead, I could pick a mother,
I wouldn't want or need another,
I wouldn't have her any other way.

There was an additional verse which didn't make it in, alluding to the fact that my mum (and her mum before her) had a historic tendency, when visiting gardens, to take a cutting to being back home and grow themselves. It didn't seem quite 'flowery' enough to include, though.

If I could pick a Primrose, I shouldn't
(Though a genetic desire
is to snip off a 'tryer',
and to take it back home in the car).

For the second little rhyme of her book, I took the Jenny Joseph poem "Warning" as a reference point. Mum did like the original "When I'm old I shall wear purple" poem, and often did (wear purple), even before she was old. So, again complete with family in-jokes and references that will mean nothing to anyone else, here's a part of the other verse I put in Mum's birthday book. I'm not including the whole thing as there are specific references to other people we know.

Now That You Can Wear Purple (after JJ)

Now that you can wear Purple,
And do what you bloody well please,
You can act like a fool
(We still think you're 'cool'),
And find some more penguins to tease!

You'll do as you feel like,
And that's why we love you,
You can do what you want, and who cares?
…
The only enigma, from straw polls we've gathered
Is purple, who'll notice the change?
From talking to friends, from what we remember
Is that you always deranged ☺

There's meercats, fire exits, and laughing till crying,
There's 'nobhead', and also 'Mad Mum,'
Wheelbarrows, 'Mum-made' cards, and broomsticks,
impressions,
For laughter you're second to none!

So though Jenny Joseph has waited
We think you are one of a kind,
Worn purple as long as you've been here,
And age is a trick of the mind.

Seeing all of the in-jokes and references I crowbarred into those lines, I realise that there are so many other little incidents that will mean nothing to anyone outside our immediate family of three, but which now form my happiest memories of Mum. There's no point in including them here as they wouldn't sound funny or interesting to you (as we frequently said when telling stories, "you had to be there"), but it is worth noting that, looking back, it is the smallest of events and snippets of conversation which bring back joy and smiles in remembering her. Just for example, there is the red and gold plastic crown we bought for her (as she always liked to joke about the Queen being a personal friend), and which we placed on her Urn for Christmas during the Queens speech the December after she died. It's a silly little tribute, but means a lot to me and my sister. There are memories of watching The Chase or Strictly (with Mum bizarrely telling me, with conviction, that Anton Du Beke was in his mid-sixties at least), afternoon napping to Pick of the Pops on a Saturday, sitting out in the back garden reading and smoking, her latter obsession with Peanut Butter Dairy Milk chocolate; but none of these memories has a 'point' it would be worth me recounting to you here. They are just some of my 'happy memories.' And you can never have too many of those.

If you're ever going through old papers and knick-knacks and think "that may as well get thrown out," think carefully about maybe keeping those things in a shoebox at the back of a wardrobe. A time may come when you'll treasure them, even if they seem insignificant to you now. The same applies after you lose someone. It was a big job clearing Mum's house afterwards, and going through all the paperwork and bits and bobs, and my sister kept a huge amount of material. I took a more practical approach (and I have a relatively small flat with no storage space) of keeping only things which held particularly strong memories. It's through my sister's cajoling that I now still have my baby bracelet giving my time of birth, as it isn't an item I initially thought I'd really have a use for, and with no-one to pass it on to. But I'm so glad now that I kept it. It links to the photos of me with Mum as a new-born and is a physical piece of the past I can look at or hold. If in doubt, keep anything that might have a meaning, for a couple of years at least.

I take after my mum in my practical side though, and two of my most treasured possessions came from her kitchen. There's a mug with a print of the New York subway system on it, which I bought her about twenty years ago, and which all her cups of tea were in, and the last remaining plate in an old dinner service; a small yellow (almost translucent by now) plate which she would eat all her main meals from. I'm sure at some point in the future they'll end up dropped or cracked but for now, they carry on being used as they were intended, and just having them in the drainer next to my other crockery, keeps Mum with me.

A last anecdote. Even in our final months, we managed to find laughter and joy in tragedy. One incident I recall made my sister and I smile, not at our Mum, but at the situation and the ridiculousness of life, which is a terrific way to look at life when the day to day grind wears you down. Find the ridiculous and smile at it. Like this one particular morning...

Mum had difficulty eating her breakfast and had brought up phlegm in the sick bowl again, so once she was settled in her chair afterwards, bowl by her feet just in case, but dozing and content, I'd popped up the road to the shops for supplies. When I got back, she'd been "sick" again, but it was sick of a suspiciously brown colour. And there were several shiny foil chocolate wrappers on the coffee table beside her in the lounge. It was no longer as scary by now when she was physically sick, as it was a regular occurrence, but I gently chided her for eating sweets when she should have eaten her healthy breakfast. Explaining as you might with a child.

"I haven't eaten any chocolates!" came the indignant response.

You know the refrain of the child with chocolate around their mouth, protesting innocence? I pointed out the brown-coloured phlegm in the sick bowl, and the several chocolate wrappers that hadn't been there when I left. Mum maintained her innocence, almost offended at the accusation, and with the rather weak excuse that she had no idea how the wrappers had got there, but she had NOT eaten chocolates! Sometimes you reach the stage where you have to laugh, and she was so serious and haughty I couldn't help myself, kissing her head and removing the litter without any further comment. I don't know if she'd completely forgotten that she'd just eaten them, or if there was an element of guilt that it had been somehow naughty, but it brought home the fibs and covering up, and the ridiculous extent they'd reached. Mum settled back with a smile; whether she thought she'd fooled me and won some sort of victory, or that I'd been mistaken, or whether there remained a portion of awareness at the ridiculousness of her claim, I don't know. But it was the sly sort of grin that told me she thought we'd won a victory.

I'll stop the random experiences and return to the narrative timeline now, of how we finally lost our mum, but I wanted those happy memories written down first, as I don't want you to think everything was sad or painful, or that there wasn't joy, right up to and including those last weeks.

At times, during the latter stages of her illness, it could feel like caring for a small child, and as I mentioned earlier, the roles of carer and cared-for were reversed from what they "should be," with your mum. And we'd reached that stage. We were also at the point where there were some more serious topics you don't or can't discuss any more, and personal situations you wouldn't admit to as they might upset her; matters around our personal lives or health which we couldn't really share with Mum. Balancing caring with regular life was next to impossible.

Looking back, I think it's better that by then Mum had reached the point where she no longer realised some of the implications of looking after her, as I know it would have hurt and upset her to think she'd in any way impacted on our 'regular lives,' but it was such a tricky balance in conversations; not to let details slip out which she might realise were because of the caring, or aspects of our self-care and health that now had to be slotted in and around our responsibilities to Mum. I wanted to try and be transparent, honest and open with her where I could, so she felt that conversations and discussions weren't hidden and that we were still able to have open, adult-to-adult discussions but at the same time, there were some things that had to be kept hidden.

By now, her health was deteriorating in a number of additional and upsetting ways. In addition to the more obvious medical problems, Mum had started to have daytime nightmares, or that was what we concluded, anyway. Napping in her chair in the lounge during the day, her face would become screwed up, sometimes her leg would kick, and she'd wake herself up, upset. She could never remember (or wouldn't say) what the dreams were, but they became more frequent. It was hard to watch. And added to our determination to spare her from any further mental stress.

I wanted to be honest with her, but the last six months of Mum's life overlapped with my own medical appointments and eventual prostate cancer diagnosis and treatment. It was only afterwards that I found out that my sister also had a similar experience at the time, and her own diagnosis.

I didn't tell Mum about the biopsy results when I was tested (I was like a bloody pin cushion and 'down there' turned black with bruising afterwards – just thought I'd share that) and while she knew I was having tests, I just couldn't admit to her what the findings meant. I didn't want to add to her concerns or upset her, and a part of me, maybe irrationally, also feared the worst and that, in the best traditions of "sod's law," Mum would manage to keep perfect recall of my tests and health, even when she forgot everything else, and she'd get distressed worrying about me.

So I tried to make light of my illness as inconsequential, and any reference to my absences would be delivered conversationally. "Oh, by the way, I won't be here Tuesday as I have more flipping tests, tshhh," or similar, so she wouldn't think I was concerned at all. I don't think Mum wanted to contemplate any other outcome either, so we both pretended there was nothing to it; and never once uttered the 'C' word itself. I'm an awkward sod in that I don't like admitting my own deep fears and insecurities (contrary to what this book might imply), so while, as you can imagine, I had a very difficult time coming to terms with my own diagnosis and the potential outcomes, the fact that we didn't need to discuss details suited me fine. I sometimes wonder how much Mum realised or guessed, but there's no way of knowing, and we both maintained the façade that it was all a bit of fuss over nothing, with me ironically falling into the trap of Mum's own approach to illness. The difference is that I decided to seek treatment, even though that had all sorts of risks because of my previous stroke history. And I did have other people I loved who I could talk to. Though being introspective, and with my 'work through the worst-case scenario' methodology in place, I preferred to go through all the what ifs in my own brain instead. Because I'm an idiot. But I'm getting off track again.

Prostate cancer is so misunderstood, though (at best), and levels and stages so varied, that I don't think Mum would have been able to follow and understand the details of my treatment and prognosis anyway, and in addition to being upset about the cancer itself, she'd have become frustrated and confused that she didn't understand the medical terminology and options. I know it would have upset her to try, and to not be able to grasp everything, so it was one of the times I was almost thankful for the dementia. And that I didn't really have the option of discussing it with her anyway.

My personal story here doesn't matter, but after several hours upside down on an operating table with robot arms playing Ker-plunk with my internal organs, my prostate was no more and I'm happy to say I'm cancer-free. And fate, for once, was relatively kind. The way timings worked out, my operation was shortly after Mum's funeral, so we got to complete everything we needed and say goodbye, and when the time came, I didn't have to worry about Mum any more, so was probably a lot more relaxed when I went under the knife. Fate isn't that kind though, and my sister needed her own operation a few months later. She too is, thankfully, cancer-free now.

We try to be positive. For both of us, having cancer found early enough allowed us to be treated and recover; Mum being spared the knowledge and worry with the timing of her death was a good thing; how the timings happened was about as positive as we could hope for. But, in both our cases, catching symptoms early was key so, whoever you are, please get yourself checked regularly. It might just save your life.

But to return to the end of this particular story...

The End

It was a Wednesday, and I'd been out of the office for an away-day in the Albert Dock with work. Although I'd called a couple of times as usual and tried to sound upbeat, Mum hadn't seemed in the most responsive of moods; her texts had been short, her talking on the phone distracted. I'd called again as I left the dock about 4pm, and it was clear to me by that point that all wasn't right. She couldn't get warm, she said, and wanted to go back to bed. That desire wasn't totally unprecedented by any means, but her tone was concerning enough that I told her I'd be over to check on her as soon as I'd had my tea.

Mum was miserable and low when I arrived, but perked up a bit as we had a cup of tea and a chat. Still complaining of being cold and tired, she repeated that she was going to bed, though. It really wasn't like her to actually get into her bed at 8 pm, and her saying she was "heading back to bed" was a constant refrain, almost joking, that we usually talked her out of. She was obviously unhappy, though, so I said fine, cancelled the bedtime carer, got her a hot water bottle, and checked on her a few times, though she soon seemed to be snoring as happily as she could.

The next morning, Mum didn't want to get up, or eat breakfast, and the carer (one of our regulars), told me she'd been out of sorts for the last couple of days. She still complained of being cold, and there was enough "not right" about her that I called out the doctor, who would arrive after lunch. I worked 'from home' at Mum's house that morning, lucky that my job allowed it, as this wasn't so common pre-COVID, and with the benefit of my company, chat, cups of tea and biscuits, Mum seemed to pick up significantly. I even joked she'd better get poorly again, now that I'd called the doctor out but, as is often the way, she was feeling much healthier when he arrived, and it looked like not much was wrong, so I thought maybe it was psychological rather than physical. He took her BP and pulse, and did a pinprick test for sepsis, but she seemed to be on the mend, so I headed back to my flat in the afternoon (as I hadn't expected to be away, so hadn't put anything in place or prepared), and my sister was due up on the Friday afternoon anyway, so it would be only 24 hours until one of us was back. In the meantime, the carers would be there as usual, four times a day, checking on her. By this stage, illness (or an "off day") wasn't unusual, so we'd passed the stage of completely panicking every time she seemed to have a bad or low spell. I spoke to Mum several times during the afternoon and evening, and she seemed better, but I was ready to head back over to her house, as I always was by then, if she went downhill.

On the Friday morning I spoke to her at breakfast, and to the carer, and she was cold once more, and said that she wanted to go back to bed, but was otherwise talking okay, about nothing in particular. The carer, one of the really good ones, could keep an eye out as she was on shift at lunchtime, and my sister would be there before teatime.

I got the call at maybe 11 am. The carer had come back early, wanting to check all was still okay, but had found Mum on the floor under the kitchen table, physically cold, and not very responsive. The one time the falls alarm should have gone off, nothing had registered, it seems. The ambulance had already been called. I got in a black cab, calling again to the carers on the way, and it seemed she'd slipped off her chair, and had probably been on the floor for an hour or more, hence her being cold, and probably in shock. I changed my destination to go straight to the hospital and meet the ambulance there.

Mum arrived just as I did, and by then was a bit embarrassed but fully awake and 'with it,' and with my sister on the way from where she lived (several hours' drive away) we talked, did crosswords, and they wheeled in different scanning machines, did several tests, and told us to stop talking, as Mum needed to save her breath. She grinned mischievously and kept whispering, and though her breathing and pulse weren't strong, she seemed fine. She went onto the ward and we were sent home at the end of visiting hours, with no particular immediate concern.

The phone call from the doctor that evening wasn't a total surprise, but hit us hard. Mum had broken her hip when she fell, and if it wasn't replaced, she'd be bedbound for the rest of her life. We didn't think she'd survive an operation, but there seemed little choice, and the doctor appeared confident and upbeat about her prospects. It was a quiet night at Mum's home, my sister and I thinking about what might come next.

The following morning we headed into the hospital, and Mum was awake, joking with us again, doing the little rhymes we always repeated, and trying a crossword, but the operation was going to be that afternoon. That was scary as shit, but everyone seemed confident and Mum herself seemed brighter and back on form, so we said we'd see her at teatime (this was when she said, "bugger off you two!"), but we were both less than convinced it would go well. Miraculously, it did seem to go smoothly, and though she was pretty out of it from the anaesthetic when we returned at teatime, she knew we were there with her, and her stats were all okay. It was a huge relief.

The next morning, the Sunday, I was planning on heading back to my flat to get some things (and we'd take shifts looking after Mum, as we had the last time she was in hospital) but I phoned at 8am, to see how she was. When we finally got through, a harassed nurse told us Mum had a good night, all was fine, and I insisted she tell Mum we were on our way in later so she didn't worry or think we'd abandoned her. As we got ready for the day, so relieved, the phone rang again about ten minutes later. Mum had taken a sudden turn for the worse, apparently, and could we come in, right away. I think we both knew. The music in the taxi on the way in, an opera aria that had a particular significance for her, was a sign to my sister of what we'd find, and when we got there, a junior doctor took us into what seemed to be an equipment cupboard (someone else was in the family room) and told us that Mum had died. We went to say goodbye to her, behind the curtain, still on the ward. The time went by in a dull and numb mindset for us.

I'm almost certain that at some point after the rounds at 7am, Mum's body had just given out, and she'd been dead by the time I'd phoned at eight; the nurse going to see and pass on our message discovering the body. But I don't like to dwell on that, and in the big scheme of things, the timeline isn't that important. The doctor had seen her on his rounds first thing in the morning, so she'd come through the night ok. She'd survived the operation and had slept comfortably. I don't want to talk any more about the rest of that day.

We try to be positive. The fact mum died before the horrors of COVID, was a strange blessing, as her passing was almost inevitably going to come within months anyway. But she hadn't been alone in an empty house at the end; she'd been warm and comfortable in a hospital bed; we'd seen her and talked after her fall; she'd joked with us; she wasn't in pain; the dementia was far enough advanced that she wouldn't have remembered the details of her fall, but not so advanced she didn't know us. Small mercies.

As I sit here writing, a couple of years on, it doesn't make me sad any more; it makes me happy to remember my mum and my times with her, even when she was ill. One sadness I do have, is of the photos in my flat; I'm starting to recognise the woman in some of them less over time. I remember the old lady, I recognise the young woman in the pictures as we've looked at so many with her; but the Mum who raised me, those photos, strangely, that Mum seems less familiar.

This ending may seem a bit rushed to you, but it was for us, and the tumble of emotions and events at the end are still the over-riding part which stays in the mind. It was over too quickly, but at the same time, mercifully quickly.

Before I move onto the fiction, which probably shows my emotions and thoughts about the whole process and legacy more than anything, I want to reiterate that this is a happy book for me, and cathartic. This chapter may have ended too quickly, and on a sad note, but that's appropriate. What came before was my memories of all the positives of my

147

mum having been alive; the jokes, the fun, the love. Mum is gone but will never be forgotten

We scattered her ashes in the village where she grew up, with big skies and rolling fields for a view, and returned her to where she belongs. The "Mum" lives on in us; the beautiful, funny, wonderful woman, has gone home.

Fiction

It's taken a while to write and put this book together and, if I'm honest, even now, I'm still not 100% certain why I did it, except perhaps that I had to.

The remainder of this book has been difficult, and is very personal to me, as it is a collection of fiction pieces I've written at various times over the last two years. I don't want to describe them up front too much, I think they should speak for themselves, but they probably show my mixed feelings and emotions more than anything in the preceding pages. Those were the facts. These are the sensations.

The poems, my Mum wouldn't have liked much (they don't rhyme and are mainly free verse) but they weren't written for her to read; they were written because I had to get them out. If you're not a fan of free verse or get put off by the very idea of 'poetry,' then just don't think of them as that at all. They're just words, thoughts, put down in a certain order to express emotions. The technicalities of scansion, rhyme-schemes, chimes, and all that bollocks, just forget it. I'm not trying to be clever or impress, just imagine these are simply the way the feelings came out of me. They weren't written for analysis or critique, just exhaled as a way of freeing the thoughts, obsessions, guilt, emotions and memories.

The act of creating and expelling the harsh thoughts is part of the healing process, and for me, doing that in private, on paper, was a way of dealing. The short story, imagining

149

one of Mum's later days, I find to be both horrible and comforting, but it helped me explore and come to terms with what I think her point of view might have been at the end, and how her daily experiences might not have been as upsetting or as traumatic as I worried they were at the time. I love you, Mum.

Reflections

Can you call yourself an orphan at fifty or
Is that too self-indulgent?

Can you excuse yourself the guilt of not succeeding
In making someone live forever?

Can you forgive yourself for the row you once had
Though you're now the only one who remembers?

Those are the easy and lighter thoughts
That don't sometimes haunt you
At two a.m.
Or make you unscrew the cap of the single malt
You only bought for special occasions.

Passing her old house and objectively critiquing the
Changes to bricks and mortar can be done without
emotion.

Talking to a photograph frame is harmless,
If done in fun;
You don't really believe your words are heard
                                    by anybody.

Watching that particular TV show
Or listening to that music
Can bring a smile or echo of a chuckle.

I'm glad those aren't the only things I remember,
They aren't the whole
Picture.
A picture needs perspective to mean more
Than just shapes and small details,
To be more than a sum of the parts.

I have a Christmas Cactus I inherited, a cutting from its constantly flowering parent cactus. Mine sits unobtrusively in the corner of my room, and stubbornly refuses to grow evenly, or to bloom. It appears healthy and happy, just does its own thing, and carries on being cactus-ey in its own way. I like that.

It will probably outlive me. I hope so.

The Empty Shell

I don't like people noticing me looking,
identifying changes,
it isn't my place to say,
what I think doesn't matter.

This isn't the house Mum lives in any more.

It still looks superficially the same,
(though I can see small differences you might not)
and my description isn't meant to be cruel.
The house isn't empty,
but it is empty of the Mum I remember.
A relative stranger lives there now.

Standing outside,
I still imagine her pottering around inside,
And imagine I can catch
a glimpse of her through a window,
even though I know it's just a shadow,
a shallow reflection.

I know it's my imagination
but what is the problem with that?
It makes it feel like my house again, too.

I know you could read these lines two ways,
and I'm ashamed I used the word shell
about one of them.
I'm also glad.

Shells are pretty, shells are unique. Hold a shell to
your ear and can hear the waves and the seaside,
and you think of holidays and childhood. Shells are
a defence for many animals, and a home for others.

A shell is a casing, a hard exterior that protects the vulnerable; its very purpose is to be that shield.

By the time you find an empty shell, the life inside has fled but it is still a thing of beauty, with every characteristic, a perfect memorial.

The Empty Shell pt.2 (Self Pity)

Who will take care of me now,
Now that you're not here?
Even when
I was looking after you,
You were looking after me,
Even then,
Just by being there.
Take care of myself? I don't know how...

Mum Hated the Dentist

My mum's mouth was a good indication of her
mental health.
Bear with me, this is going somewhere.

She had a plate, false teeth,
And after her second spell in hospital,
The long one,
They scrubbed that plate so completely,
Sent it home with her for a fresh start,
Pink and white and clean.
Clinically correct.
Just not the same.

Like your lungs, post smoking, I'm guessing the
plate just didn't feel right, and I could see you didn't
like how it felt. Because you wouldn't see a dentist
for twenty years, it must already have been tight
and ill fitting, but it had been on your terms before
they scraped it clean and fresh, without asking you
first.

There weren't many teeth left at the end, and I know
you 'helped' one or two of the wobbly ones on the
way yourself; better that than having to see the
dentist. You protested that you hadn't done that, of
course.

Fibbing and covering up
Denial
Putting up with the problems hoping they'd go away
Avoidance
Never wanting to admit how scared you were

I see a parallel anyway.

We'd always put the tablet in your denture pot for you, because that's how you protect them, and because you'd stopped bothering. You just didn't see the point. You were so tired I know, my lovely.

And you didn't like looking at the dentures, did you? A reminder of the teeth that had gone, a time before. Pink and glistening, they didn't even seem like a part of you. So best ignore them.

Out of sight, out of mind.

Snapshots

There are nine pictures of my mother, in frames in
my flat,
On display on four different bookcases.
These aren't posed or professional,
And ages range from her twenties to her eighties.
I can see her life.

There are only two of my dad,
But he'd been dead when seven of the Mum ones
were taken,
So the ratio is even and fair,
Based on the timeline
Alone.

There are nine pictures of my mum
And Mum is in eight of them,
The ninth has an old lady who looks exactly like my
Mum
From the outside.

The two in which she's laughing,
open mouthed,
not caring about the camera
are my favourites.

Is nine (pictures) too many?
I frankly couldn't give a fuck what you think.

Has The Lady Been Yet?

The light shone through the chink she'd left in my curtains, but they were thin enough that my room was never dark after dawn. I blinked slowly, a pleasant buzz coming from my right as I yawned. I didn't know how many times I'd woken during the night, but that didn't matter now. I felt tired but was quite awake. I must have slept well. I realised that it was music from my radio to the right, and I felt comfortable hearing the tune. I didn't know it, but it sounded familiar. I yawned again, my brow crinkling slightly. I don't think it had been a nice dream, but I didn't want to try and remember that. It hadn't been a good night but it was over now, and it was the daytime. I closed my eyes again, just for a second.

I hadn't heard the back door open but was suddenly aware of noises outside my bedroom. I tensed and then relaxed almost at the same time; another person was meant to be here now. A bright voice called through, "Good Morning, Liz" and I turned my head as a woman in a light blue uniform dress came through the door. I knew that I knew her, but couldn't recall her actual name. She smiled at me and told me it was a beautiful day, as she pulled back the curtains, letting the daylight stream in fully. I blinked as she busied herself around, doing whatever it was she did.

"And how are we today?"

I couldn't really not reply so I smiled, and said I was just going to have five more minutes. She laughed, saying that I

159

must be "on form" today, whatever that meant. Then she sat on the edge of my bed and started asking me what I had planned for such a beautiful morning.

"I think I'll go to the beach, and then maybe Venice... and then watch The Chase."

I don't know where the words came from but she smiled, "Same as yesterday then, maybe Rome today instead? Shall we get up?"

The lady pulled back my duvet gently and I automatically put my arm out to the side of the bed, and after a moment, put it back again. For some reason she had a sad smile, as she said she'd help me. It was a struggle today. She'd asked if I'd wanted the frame, and I'd said I didn't need it, but accepted it anyway and she stood behind me as we headed through to the bathroom.

Back sitting on my bed, half dressed, she chattered away, though I wasn't really taking it in yet, and she kneeled to rub cream into my legs. I don't know why she did that, but I let her as it seemed to make her happy, and I looked out of the window at the blossom on the tree. Towards it, anyway; I couldn't really see the detail from where I sat.

"Have you answered that yet, Lizzy?"

She put my mobile phone in my hand, returning to rubbing the cream in, and I smiled. Who'd have ever thought I'd have a mobile phone, who'd have thought there would even be such a thing, but I wouldn't be without it. I wasn't even aware I'd flipped it open, or pressed to read the message, which was from someone named Kit. He texted me every morning, didn't he? I smiled. I reached for my glasses so I didn't have to strain, and read the full message, using the down button to track to the end. He said it was a

160

beautiful sunny day, but he didn't want to work so was going back to bed. I gave a little laugh. He always said that. I texted '*me 2. The lady here, rubbing my legs*' and hit send. I felt better. It was strange that people had trouble with mobile phones. I found them easy.

The handset beeped again as I was sitting at the table, cup of hot tea in front of me and the paper waiting to be read. I picked it up and opened it. The lady was in the kitchen, sorting my Weetabix, which was nice of her. I frowned at the tea and put the phone down. It wasn't really milky enough, but tea was tea, and it would be rude to complain when she'd made it for me. I opened the paper, unfolding it, and looked at the cover, not really interested in what was there.

"Was that Sarah?"

The lady came through with my cereal and a bag of pills, which I eyed suspiciously. I looked at her blankly.

"The phone, Lizzie, I heard it go; was that your daughter?"

I picked the handset up again and flipped it open but there wasn't a message showing so I put it back down and reached for my spoon.

"It sometimes doesn't show as new if you've opened it, you remember, you told me that yesterday?"

If she knew that, I must have said it I suppose, and she flipped the thing back open and pressed a button or two, handing it over to me. '*Ello. Just on walk to work. Warm but overcast. Who's there with you this morning?*' Yes, there had been two texts, two children, that was right. I glanced at the lady fiddling with the pills. I knew she came a lot, but wasn't sure what her name was, and it would be rude to ask now;

she obviously knew me well. So I decided to ignore the question. I concentrated on tapping out my reply. '*Just avin brekkie.*'

It had been hard to get one of the pills down today and I coughed a lot, but the lady kept insisting I drink some water so in the end I did, to shut her up, and I soon got over the coughing. She was talking about *Strictly*, and I suddenly remembered the funny dance from the man who'd gone out in this week's programme, and we talked about that for a few minutes, before she went to do something in the bedroom. I unfolded the paper again, glasses on, tea half-drunk and was feeling far more 'with it' as my mobile rang. It was my son, on his way to work. He sounded bright and breezy, and reminded me he would be over tomorrow night, which I told him would be lovely, and I really meant it. It was so much easier when someone was here who you didn't have to pretend with, and who would look after you. He told me something about work, and we talked for several minutes. He asked me who was with me today and I told him it was Emily, not wanting to admit I'd forgotten her name momentarily. He said he thought it was supposed to be Fran, and could he have a word with her, about the schedule. Of course it was Fran. I'd known that. I shouted out to Fran that Kit wanted a word, holding out the phone so he could ask whatever it was he needed to ask. I don't know what they said to each other but I stuck my tongue out at her as she told him I was on good form today. Not in a mean way - joking. I knew she enjoyed me doing that, like I was a child. She chuckled and told him what I was doing, which pleased me. Then she went into the kitchen with the phone and I flipped through the pages, pausing on a photo of Anton Du

Beck and a story about a chat show he was going to be on. The lady came back and handed me the phone and the man on the other end said he was in work now, so would speak to me later.

"See you soon, love you lots!"

Kit always said that when we finished a conversation, too. I said it back, and he hung up. Fran called through.

"He said Sarah was coming this weekend, that'll be nice, won't it?"

I nodded and agreed, though I wasn't really sure what she meant.

I was nodding off again, sat in my chair in the front room, paper on my lap and cup of tea and glass of water on the side table, walking frame in front of me, hot water bottle at my side. It was a warm morning and the paper hadn't held my attention. "Come on Liz, get a grip of yourself," I told myself out loud, shuffling to get comfortable and reaching for the crossword book and pen on the coffee table. The phone was flashing, which meant I had a message, so I opened it and answered my friend from two doors away, who was going shopping, but I messaged that I didn't need anything. She texted back again that she'd call round later, so I sipped my water and picked up the newspaper.

I was sitting at the table with my newspaper, reading about Anton du Beck when the lady came in, so it must have been lunchtime already. I wasn't really hungry, but she came every day. She smiled and said hello, and how had my morning been? I didn't recognise this one, but it was the same blue uniform, and she seemed very friendly, so I asked how her morning had been, too. She said something I didn't catch, and asked me if I wanted a cuppa, which of course I did, you can never have enough cups of tea, and she noticed the newspaper open. She said something about *Strictly* from last week and I agreed, and we talked about the upcoming Blackpool show, and who we thought would go out, as she asked me what I wanted for dinner. I told her I wasn't that hungry, and would make something myself later, but she insisted, said I had to eat something with my pills. She laughed when I suggested I could just not have the pills as I didn't really need them. I wasn't really sure what they were for, to be honest, but I was supposed to keep taking them. She called out what was in the fridge and I agreed to have a cheese sandwich. The phone rang while she was in the kitchen and it was my son, Kit, on his way back for his own lunch. I smiled to myself as he talked and asked him when he was coming next. I didn't want to sound like I was pressuring him, but it would be lovely to see him again. He said tomorrow, and that he'd be here after work, and said he was going to warm a quiche for his own lunch, asking what I was having. I said a sandwich and asked what time he would be coming, and he said after tea, so probably about half-past six. He said I should ask Fran to check if he needed to bring any teabags, as I might be getting low, so I shouted the question to her, using her name, so he knew I was talking to her. She was very nice and said we had plenty, so I repeated the message and he said some things about work. He said he'd let me go and have my lunch, and said the "see you soon, love you lots" again, which I repeated back.

Fran came through with the tea and sandwiches, and I told her that he was coming tomorrow. I added a story I'd remembered about when he was little and had once got up in the night and peed in the fridge. Fran laughed and talked about her kids as well while she sorted my pills and gave me a glass of water to take them with. I don't know how long we chatted for, it was lovely, though she did keep nudging me to eat, so I took a small bite to placate her. Fran said she'd just run the hoover round and I told her there was no need, but she seemed to want to and wouldn't take no for an answer, so I went through to the lounge. She brought the sandwich plate and put it on the table next to me, making me lift my legs as she hoovered, and we laughed at that. She seemed a very happy girl. I remembered that she was going to France soon with her kids, so asked about that and she stopped hoovering to tell me. I caught her looking at my uneaten cheese sandwich, and she asked if I wanted a biscuit with my tea. I grinned; Fran knew me quite well. She tidied round and fussed and asked if I was doing anything when my daughter came up at the weekend. I hadn't known Sarah was coming, or I might have forgotten, so I said we'd do a lot of crosswords and watch *Strictly* together. I loved having company watching my shows and discussing them. And she loved crosswords as much as I did, must be in the genes. I was really looking forward to her being here. The ladies were lovely, but it was so much nicer just me and the kids. I say kids, but they're all grown up now. I frowned to myself. They shouldn't need to come and see me so much, as lovely as it was. They had their own lives. I remember looking after my dad when he got old and confused, and how hard it had been for everyone. I hoped I would never get to that stage.

I hadn't realised Fran had been talking, and with a promise I'd eat my sandwich in a bit, she asked if I wanted a bottle (hot water) and I said yes please. As she was in the kitchen, my mind drifted back to looking after Dad. It had been so sad, seeing him like that, and it had been months after Mum had died that we all had to take care of him. I didn't really pay attention as the lady came back in with my hot water bottle and glass of water, and said she'd see me tomorrow. That would be nice.

My phone went again about one, and it was Sarah, waiting for the bus as she had the afternoon off. She asked if the lady had been yet, and who it was, and I couldn't recall her name so I said Tina, I thought, as I knew that was one of them. Then she fussed, asking what I'd had for lunch, so I told her I'd had a sandwich and some crisps, but she kept pushing and asked what sort of sandwich. I was a bit flustered and wasn't sure what it had been but I told her ham, as that was likely enough, but she said I didn't have any ham in, so it must have been something else, could I remember what? I must admit I snapped at her a little, telling her to stop getting at me. Sometimes my daughter treated me like I was a child. There was an awkward silence for a moment, and she asked if I wanted anything bringing when she came up at the weekend. I asked her what time she was coming and she said she'd be here before eight if the traffic was good. That would be nice. We could listen to *Friday Night is Music Night* on Radio 2. For some reason, she seemed delighted I'd said that, and nattered about some of the people at her work for a few minutes before she said her bus was coming. Then she said the "see you soon, love you lots" too, and I said it back. It was a nice little ritual we had, always saying that on the phone. I can't remember why we'd started it, but it was a nice last thing to say to someone.

I'd had an uneasy nap in the afternoon, nasty dreams, and I drank my water and went to make myself a cup of tea and to refill my hot water bottle. I wasn't helpless, I was quite capable, and sometimes I think people forgot that. I chuckled as I grabbed the frame and pulled myself to my feet. My son was always horrified by the way I poured the boiling water into the bottle from the kettle, but it was hardly complicated. I'd been doing it since before he was born. I put my cup on the table on the way past and carried on towards the bathroom for a wee, wondering what my neighbour was up to today, she usually called round.

When I settled myself again, moving the plate with the sandwich to make room for my cup of tea, it took an age to get comfy, and get my position right. I eyed the plate suspiciously. I don't think I was supposed to touch it, and, I think the lady might get upset if I threw it into the food bin, so I left it there and put the TV on, it would be my quiz shows soon. That was when I heard my friend call through from the back door. I sighed and struggled to my feet, calling out a hello back. It was nice to have visitors, but they always seemed to come when I was getting settled for a nap.

I woke with a start, another nasty dream I think, but I wasn't sure what. I bit my lip, feeling a bit jittery, and reached for my tea, which was cold, but I sipped at it anyway. The TV was noisy and distracting so I reached for the remote to turn it down, or off, muttering to myself and telling no-one in particular that I wished it would just

167

bugger off. I must have been doing something wrong though, and nothing happened. I pressed again and tried some of the other buttons, but nothing seemed to work. I felt stupid, like there was something obvious I should be doing, but nothing I tried worked, and the TV was so loud and distracting. I clenched my fingers several times, pushing up my glasses and trying the buttons again, but nothing worked. I think I started to panic a bit, as whatever I did, I couldn't turn it off, and I had to turn it off. It was a stupid, simple thing and I couldn't do it. But I had to, I had to turn it off. I refused to be beaten, and even though I know my hands were shaking a bit I reached for my mobile phone. I never seem to have trouble with that one bit of technology so I texted my son, just a short message '*can't seem to turn tv off.*' I didn't want to worry him, but I knew he'd be able to fix it for me. I sniffed and rubbed a tear from the corner of my eye, trying once again with the remote. Just as I knew it would, my phone rang a minute later, though it still made me jump. He said hello and asked what the problem was with the TV and I tried to keep my voice sounding calm, laughed, and said I was probably just being silly, but I couldn't turn the volume down or off. I tried to concentrate on what he was saying, but the noise of the television was so distracting. Yes, of course I had the right remote. He described it to me and what he said matched the thing in my left hand, so I followed what he told me to do; carefully point it at the bottom of the screen and press the big green button. I did everything he said but it still wasn't working. He said it was okay, and kept talking as I put the remote down and sipped at my cold tea again, phone pressed to my ear, straining to hear him over the sounds of the man on the television. My son said he was working from memory, but hold it up and try pressing the red button. I didn't hear what he said after that as I lifted my right hand to look closely, like he told me, and pressed the big red button. Then I put the phone back to my ear but it was silent, and I kept saying hello but he'd gone. He wouldn't have left without saying goodbye so it must be yet another technology problem, but that just made things worse. There was a loud advert about a kitchen on, and he was gone and I was on my own and didn't know what to do. I just sat, looking at my lifeless mobile phone and trying not to cry. I jumped when it rang again, and fumbled to answer.

"I don't know what to do, it's broken and won't work and I did what you said and it's so loud. I'm sorry, I'm really sorry but I don't know what to do."

I apologised and told him what was happening again and again, and could make out a buzzing like someone else was talking and then it got louder. "Mum... Mum... MUM... MUM! Just listen... LISTEN TO ME... JUST LISTEN... ITS OKAY... I'm sorry, are you listening? It will be fine, I promise. It isn't a big problem, is it? The TV is still on is all that's happened, and the lady will be here soon and if we can't fix it now then she can do that when she arrives. Just take a deep breath, love. And again. Are you listening?"

His voice came properly into focus as he'd started to talk, and I forced myself to listen. Just the sound of his voice was soothing, calming me, letting me know it was okay and that things would be fine. I took a breath. I knew I was being silly but it had all just got a bit much for a moment. I said I was listening, and that I was sorry.

169

"Pick up the remote again in your free hand... the BIG LONG BLACK ONE, not your phone... have you got it, are you still listening, love? I'm really sorry I was shouting, I just needed to get your attention."

I hadn't noticed he'd been shouting, and I did what he told me to, confirming each step, and calming down, feeling just a little bit sillier for making such a fuss. I slid the battery compartment down at the back, and rolled the batteries round with my thumb like he said, then put it back on and slowly pointed the remote, and the TV switched off. I don't know why, but it was such a relief I almost cried again. He said something about making the lady check when she came, and that he was looking forward to seeing me tomorrow. It would be so good to have him here. I didn't like to tell him but I don't think I panicked the same when he was here. I didn't want to make a fuss, but couldn't help telling him how lovely it would be to have him here. He made some jokes about the train, and said he had to go, but would call me again when he was walking home, if I was sure I was okay? I told him I'd be fine, and I was sorry for making a fuss, and we did the "see you soon, love you lots" line again, which felt really nice, and familiar. I went for a wee, then came back through and got comfy again, putting the TV on for *Tipping Point*.

The lady came earlier than usual, which meant earlier tea, but that was okay. It was Nicola, I knew this one's name, as she was always happy and called me "my lovely," rather than by my name. She asked how my day was, as I got to my feet and used my frame to go through to the table, and I told her the truth; nothing special, no visitors today. As I sat down, she came back from the lounge with raised eyebrows, my undrunk tea and uneaten sandwich plate in her hands.

"You have to try and eat something, lovely. I'll get into awful trouble with your son and daughter if you keep leaving things untouched."

"I won't tell if you won't!"

I grinned, and she chuckled and told me I was incorrigible, but I had to agree to have something proper for my tea, and eat it. And did I want a cuppa? I said okay, and was thirsty for a proper cup of tea. Nicola always made it just the way I liked it; I don't know how she knew. I went back for the paper, to show her the story about *Strictly*, and we chatted, and I said I'd like egg and chips, and a piece of walnut cake. She laughed and said fine, and I was actually looking forward to that. I was a bit peckish. I was quite capable of making my own food, but Kit said the ladies were there to do it, so I should let them, and enjoy being waited on.

Depending on who you got, it was usually fine, but I liked Nicola in particular. My son phoned while the chips were cooking, as he walked home, and he asked how I was doing. I'll be honest, I was a bit distracted talking to Nicola, so I just said yes to whatever he said. He seemed very pleased when I told him Nicola was making me egg and chips though. He laughed and asked if I was having cake as well and I joked that, "I might..."

He asked to have a word with her and I handed the phone over, flicking through my paper as they talked for a minute, and she headed into the lounge to do something, then back to the kitchen, and to the lounge. She passed the phone back and I told him my tea was almost ready and we said our "see you soon..." goodbyes. As she buttered the bread, Nicola told me she'd changed the batteries in the TV remote, and said Kit had told her I'd had a bit of trouble with them. "Not really..." I didn't remember them being a problem but if he said so, it had probably been something and nothing and I'd put it out of my mind. We talked for ages, as she washed up and tidied, and said she'd be back in the morning, but Fran was coming tonight at bedtime. I really liked that she kept calling me "my lovely," and it was over too fast. I wanted to ask if she'd like to stay longer, but I know she had a job to go to. She went to a gentleman a few miles away after me on a Wednesday. She always came Wednesday teatime, Nicola.

I was happily settled back in my chair with my bottle and tea before the end of *The Chase*, and my eyes were just starting to droop when my phone went, the landline this time. Someone had put it on the table next to me to save me getting up, and it was my daughter ringing, who said she'd not heard back from her texts. I didn't remember getting any but she was right, the light was flashing on the mobile, so I looked as she talked. Just the usual, how our days were, that nothing much had happened. The usual, but it was really nice. Then she asked me if the lady had been yet and I said no, not yet. I wasn't sure of the time but I knew someone would come eventually, so I don't know why she fussed. She asked if I was sure and I said I didn't know, and changed the subject, asking if she'd be here in time for *Friday Night Is Music Night* when she drove up. I always worried when she drove, it was such a long way, but she said she should be up in time, and I smiled at that. It would be really nice to listen to it with her, and maybe do a crossword, or talk about the holidays we'd been on. We did that now and again, and I usually remembered lots of details, which was surprising as some of it was quite a while ago.

It was quite a long evening. There was nothing much on telly, so I just read the rest of my paper, and did a crossword or two. Kit and Sarah texted a few times, once about a documentary one of them thought I'd like which was on ITV, so I put it on but it didn't hold my attention. I may have nodded off a little. My sister texted, which was really nice, and I texted back, telling her that Kit was coming tomorrow and Sarah on Friday. I had a notepad by the chair, that I jotted some of these things down on, with a little book of instructions the kids had written; how to search for phone messages when the phone didn't beep, how to get answerphone messages, things like that. It was very nice of them but I didn't need the instructions and they lived permanently somewhere under one of my magazines. I did the crossword in my TV guide, and read a couple of articles in it, but the lady arrived before I noticed. I didn't even hear her get the key and come in. She was familiar but I didn't know this one's name. She made me a cup of tea and asked if I wanted cheese and crackers, which I always did. She cut the cheese a bit thick but I forced myself to eat it, as it would be rude to complain about such a silly thing.

She talked a lot, and fluttered round doing things, then brought through my pyjamas. She helped me get changed and put cream on my legs (I don't know why, but they always seem to do that), talking about her kids and a holiday they were going on. I don't know why I couldn't remember her name earlier, but the holiday thing reminded me; it was

Fran. She asked if I wanted the bottle to warm my bed and sat with me a while, chatting, and asking if I wanted to go through now, but I said I was going to stay up and read my paper for a while; it was a bit early for bed. She left about nine forty-five; I know because I looked at the clock, sighing that it was still so early. I picked up my puzzle book and put on my glasses.

Kit texted about quarter past ten, to say he was going to head to bed himself as he had an early start, but he was looking forward to seeing me tomorrow, adding 'Yeeeeyyyy! :-D xxx.' It would be so nice to have him here. I wondered absently when Sarah was coming next as I texted back that I was heading to bed too, and 'nighty night.' I put the phone down and picked up my puzzle book. I knew I was putting off going to bed, but I didn't like it. I didn't mind the routine; lights off, check the door locked, wee, and the lady would already have pulled the curtains and put the clothes out for morning, put a glass of water by my bed and had put my teeth in the tray for me before she'd gone. It was the being in bed, lying down, that I didn't like. I'd have Radio 2 on, of course, but would lie awake, not able to get comfy, part of me knew I would. And probably get a bit scared, being silly, worrying I might not wake up again. I did it every night before telling myself to stop being stupid and go to sleep. I tried not to think about it, as it would only make me antsy.

It was unusual no-one had texted to say goodnight, so I thought I'd stay up a little longer in case a message came through.

Closure

I wrote this final poem two years after Mum died, shortly before visiting the location where we'd scattered her ashes. It's an indication of where I am now, reconciled.

The Cricket Pitch

The sky is broad and limitless here,
The undulations gentle,
Cowed and unrailed.

She never tires of the patchwork jigsaw,
So many greens,
The flat and the leafed,
So many greys and whites,
Coddling the blue.

So many memories permeate again,
From the paths and fields and air itself.
Home brings every one back.

Every so often, there is the sound of willow,
The low of the cattle watching,
The smattering of polite applause,
And a wicked generational cackle on the wind.

No body recalls arriving,
But distantly she knows
That all that matter will return to her
In good time.

She is in no rush now.

Afterword

Today is Mother's Day, 2022, which seemed appropriate for writing this concluding section, as I didn't want to end this book on what some might see as a negative. I'll be honest, the short story really was unpleasant for me to write, but I think that's important to acknowledge. As a carer, you can never know what might be going on in the mind of someone suffering from dementia, and there are times when you imagine the worst-case scenario, but who is it the worst for? If thoughts like those I wrote went through Mum's mind, it's an awful thing for me to imagine, but from her point of view, there's no lingering on the negative, no lasting upset or trauma; she dealt with the days moment by moment, and might have wondered why a few things were happening, but knew she was safe and cared for. If some of her days were like that, it might upset me, but the only important thing, really, was her happiness and safety. And I retain the memory of two Mums. One is in those later days, when we were the 'grown-ups,' sometimes making the difficult calls, but the other is of the Mum who raised me, and the line between the two overlaps.

I can't pretend it was an easy period, or that I don't wish things had happened differently, but even through the grim times and illnesses there was joy, happiness and laughter, and a hell of a lot of hugs. One of the nicer things is that, as a carer, I got to be a child again too, playing games, listening to kids' songs, making silly jokes, and most of all, giving and getting a lot of hugs and love. That was the beauty of pre (and post) COVID caring. I'll never know how much Mum remembered, or was aware of, or really understood, in those last months, but if she remembered anything, I suspect it was the laughter, hugs and fun.

This has been difficult to write and remember, but I said at the beginning I think it might be cathartic, and it has been. Finding an outlet for admitting the worries and thoughts you have (and wish you didn't), writing anecdotes and history, is easy. But nothing can totally prepare you for the experience (and aftermath) of something like this. But if you are caring for someone with dementia, I hope some of this chimes true, and you know you're not alone; if you have friends going through the same thing, it might help you to understand what the family are going through, and if you're likely to embark on this journey yourself, I hope there will be a few pointers and thoughts, and a realisation that there is no 'right' way to cope or act, and consequently no 'wrong' ways either.

And there is always hope. That unexpected smile, joke, anecdote from the person you're caring for, are like a break in the clouds and a beam of pure joy that makes it all worthwhile. It was never about me, it was about looking after my mum, and her safety, contentment, and my sister and I making sure she knew how much she was loved. You can never know what's going on inside, but I hope Mum retained that knowledge throughout, and knew we did our absolute best. She raised us, loved us, sacrificed for us, and being there for whatever she needed was the very least we could do.

There's a famous Teddy Kennedy saying that I'd like to mis-quote, if you'll allow mu indulgence: "Never say in grief you are sorry she's gone. Rather, say in thankfulness you are grateful she was here."

And I'll end by saying this one final time, because you can never say the words too many times.

I love you Mum xxx

Novels by Kit Derrick

The Raven Sound -   978-1-8384267-0-5 - ebook
                                978-1-8384267-2-9 - paperback

Man In The Bath -   978-1-8384267-1-2 - ebook
                                  978-1-8384267-3-6 - paperback

tEXt me -   978-1-8384267-4-3 - ebook
                                  978-1-8384267-5-0 - paperback

Hope Is A Six Letter Word -
                                  978-1-8384267-6-7 - ebook
                                  978-1-8384267-7-4 - paperback

Contact Details

www.kitderrick.com

Twitter @Kitderrick1

Printed in Great Britain
by Amazon